Contents

AF737557

List of editors, author and collaborators

Editors

Harald Ostensen M.D., Coordinator, Team for Diagnostic Imaging and Laboratory Technology, WHO, Geneva, Switzerland

Holger Pettersson M.D., Professor of Radiology, Lund University, Sweden, Co-chairman, The Global Steering Group for Education and Training in Diagnositic Imaging, Director, The WHO Collaborating Centre for Training and Education in Diagnostic Imaging, Lund, Sweden

Author

Staffan Sandström M.D., Consultant radiologist, Head of the Pediatric Section, Department of Radiology, King Fahd National Guard Hospital (KFNGH), Riyadh, Saudi Arabia, Senior Consultant, The WHO Collaborating Centre for Education and Training in Radiology, Lund University Hospital, Lund, Sweden

Collaborators

K. Åkerman R.T., Hôpital de Panzi, Bukavu, DR Kongo

T. Chakera M.D., Royal Perth Hospital, Australia

P. Corr M.D., University of Natal, South Africa

K. Eklund R.T., Lund University Hospital, Lund, Sweden

L. Frostgård R.T., Lund University Hospital, Lund, Sweden

C. Fyledal-Kastberg R.T., Lund University Hospital, Lund, Sweden

R. Garcia Monaco M.D., Hospital Italiano de Buenos Aires, Argentina

R. Günther M.D., Technical University of Aachen, Germany

T. Holm M.D., Lund University Hospital, Lund, Sweden

V. Jackson M.D., Indiana University School of Medicine, Indianapolis, IN, USA

M. Joshi M.D., LTMG Hospital, Bombay, India

P. Palmer M.D., University of California, Davis, CA, USA

M. Watnick M.D., Noble Hospital, Westfield, MA, USA

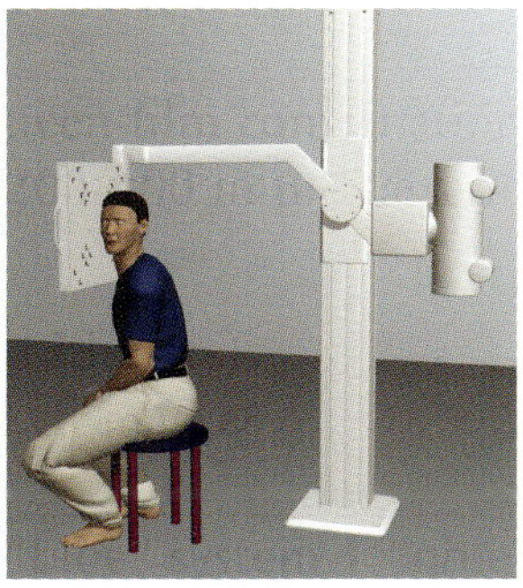
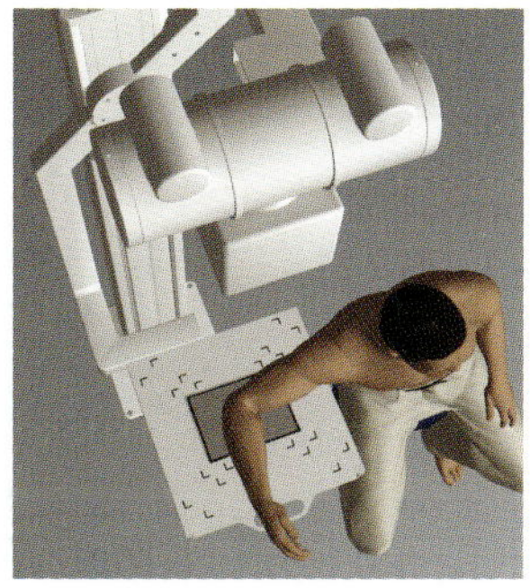
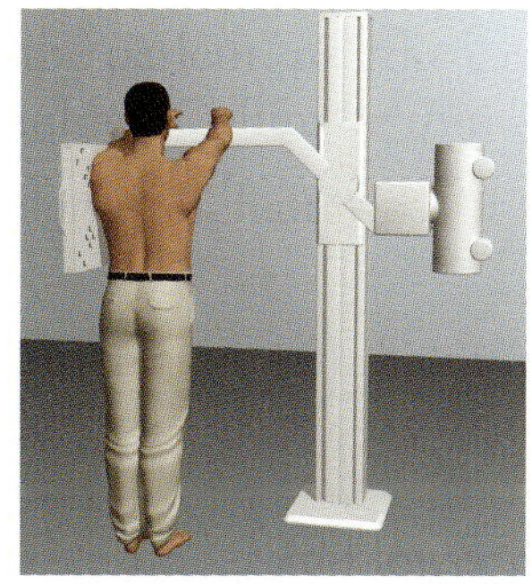

The WHO manual of diagnostic imaging

Radiographic Technique and Projections

Editors

Harald Ostensen M.D.

Holger Pettersson M.D.

Author

Staffan Sandström M.D.

In collaboration with

K. Åkerman R.T., T. Chakera M.D., P. Corr M.D., K. Eklund R.T., L. Frostgård R.T., C. Fyledal-Kastberg R.T., R. Garcia Monaco M.D., R. Günther M.D., T. Holm M.D., V. Jackson M.D., M. Joshi M.D., P. Palmer M.D., M. Watnick M.D.

Published by the World Health Organization in collaboration with the International Society of Radiology

WHO Library Cataloguing-in-Publication Data

Sandström, Staffan.

The WHO manual of diagnostic imaging : radiographic technique and projections / Staffan Sandström ; editors Harald Ostensen, Holger Pettersson.

(WHO manual of diagnostic imaging)

1.Diagnostic imaging – manual 2.Radiography – manual I.Ostensen, Harald II.Pettersson, Holger III.Title VI.Series

ISBN 92 4 154608 5 (NLM classification: WN 180)

© World Health Organization 2003

All rights reserved. Publications of the World Health Organization can be obtained from Marketing and Dissemination, World Health Organization, 20 Avenue Appia, 1211 Geneva 27, Switzerland (tel: +41 22 791 2476; fax: +41 22 791 4857; email: bookorders@who.int). Requests for permission to reproduce or translate WHO publications – whether for sale or for noncommercial distribution – should be addressed to Publications, at the above address (fax: +41 22 791 4806; email: permissions@who.int).

The designations employed and the presentation of the material in this publication do not imply the expression of any opinion whatsoever on the part of the World Health Organization concerning the legal status of any country, territory, city or area or of its authorities, or concerning the delimitation of its frontiers or boundaries. Dotted lines on maps represent approximate border lines for which there may not yet be full agreement.

The mention of specific companies or of certain manufacturers' products does not imply that they are endorsed or recommended by the World Health Organization in preference to others of a similar nature that are not mentioned. Errors and omissions excepted, the names of proprietary products are distinguished by initial capital letters.

The World Health Organization does not warrant that the information contained in this publication is complete and correct and shall not be liable for any damages incurred as a result of its use.

Designed and typeset in Sweden
Printed in India

Foreword

Modern diagnostic imaging offers a vast spectrum of modalities and techniques, which enables us to study the function and morphology of the human body in details that approaches science fiction.

However, it should be noted that even in the most advanced Imaging Department in the economically privileged parts of the world, 70–80% of all clinically relevant questions may be solved by using the two main *cornerstones* of diagnostic imaging, which are Radiography (X-ray) and Ultrasonography.

It should also be remembered that thousands of hospitals and institutions worldwide do not have the facilities to perform even these fundamental imaging procedures, for lack of equipment and/or diagnostic imaging skills.

Therefore, WHO in collaboration with the International Commission for Radiologic Education (ICRE) of the International Society of Radiology (ISR) is creating a series of "*WHO Manuals of Diagnostic Imaging*", developed under the umbrella of the Global Steering Group for Education and Training in Diagnostic Imaging. Among the members of this group are the major regional and global societies involved in Diagnostic Imaging, including the International Society of Radiology (ISR), the International Society of Radiographers and Radiological Technologists (ISRRT), and the World Federation for Ultrasound in Medicine and Biology (WFUMB).

The full series of manuals will primarily cover the examination techniques and interpretation of Radiography, in a later stage also Ultrasonography. The manuals are meant for health care personnel who in their daily work are responsible for producing and interpreting radiographs, be they radiologists or other medical specialists, general practitioners, or radiological technologists working in rural areas.

The manuals are authored by authorities in the specific fields dealt with within each manual, and supported by a group of collaborators who together cover the experience, knowledge and needs, which are specific for different regions of the world.

It is our sincere hope that the manuals will prove helpful in the daily routine, facilitating the diagnostic work up and hence the treatment, to the best benefit for the patient and it is with great pleasure and anticipation we present to you, the readers, the next manual in this series: "*Radiographic Technique and Projections*".

Geneva, Switzerland and Lund, Sweden, May 2003

Harald Ostensen
Holger Pettersson

Preface

This manual on radiographic technique and projections, is a successor to the *Manual of Radiographic Technique* that was published in 1986 with Drs T Holm, P Palmer and E Lehtinen as authors, and was meant as a manual for the WHO Basic Radiological System—WHO-BRS. The present manual can be used with any equipment, but is especially designed for the use with X-ray machines that comply with the specifications for the World Health Organization Imaging System for Radiology, WHIS-RAD.

The *positioning* of the patient is illustrated with a computed animation technique, showing one male and one female patient that are meant to represent all ethnic groups in the world. Reasonable *cassette-screen-film combinations* are suggested, as well as *exposure values*, which have to be adjusted to local conditions. Each page contains a short recommendation of how to handle the patient, and it should, as a rule, be possible to perform the examination of the patient only following the illustrations and instructions on the relevant page. An acceptable, usually normal, *resulting X-ray image* is shown. Following the instructions, the result will be a standard projection that is easily repeated for comparison and easily understood by physicians and others trained to interpret radiographs.

The work with this manual has been done at the WHO Collaborating Centre in Lund, with the old BRS manual as base, and with a strong support from the whole Department of Diagnostic Imaging at the Lund University Hospital, as well as with input from members of the ISRRT and members of the International Commission on Radiologic Education (ICRE). The important input from Dr Thure Holm and Dr Philip Palmer should be noted. The devoted and highly professional and skillful work of the department photographer, Göran Eliasson, should be specifically acknowledged, and so should the work with the final lay-out, performed by Dr Kaj Knutson.

Lund and Riyadh, May 2003

Staffan Sandström

General principles for good radiographic practice

Equipment

Appropriate equipment, well maintained, is the basis for all good radiographic practice.

The present manual is primarily meant for the WHIS-RAD system (the World Health Imaging System for Radiology), but with appropriate modifications the instructions may be used with any type of adequate radiographic machines.

For a detailed description of the WHIS-RAD system, see page 113.

Maintenance and management

It is mandatory for good radiographic practice that the examination room with its X-ray equipment and accessories, as well as the dark room and the facilities to evaluate radiographs are in good condition. For a thorough description of management and maintenance, see the WHO Manual "Quality Assurance Work Book", Geneva 2001. (WHO/DIL/01.3)

Patient care

A radiographic examination is an integrated part of clinical management and care of a patient, and the same rules for good patient care apply for the radiographic personnel as for the rest of the clinical team.

Always give each patients a friendly greeting, treat them with care and respect their individuality.

Observe the medical/clinical instructions (concerning the patient's mobility, possible medication, etc.), given by the referring doctor.

Always make sure that the films are marked with correct name of the patient, date and name of the hospital.

And always remember: a professional, well-performed examination is good patient care.

Radiation protection

X-rays are potentially harmful, and should be used with care.

Care for the personnel and persons accompanying the patient:

- stand behind the control panel when the X-ray exposure is made.
- make sure that lead aprons are worn if the patient needs to be held.
- if possible, do not allow anyone else in the X-ray room. If other persons must be present, keep them behind the control panel when the exposure is made.
- when supplied, always wear your film badge. Have it checked regularly.

Care for the patient:

The radiation risk for the patients being x-rayed is very low because they are exposed to x-rays infrequently, and because only a small part of the body is exposed for each patient. Therefore, whenever there is a clinical reason for X-ray examination such an examination is justified and should be performed. However, always try to get all the details right the first time, so that there is no need for a second exposure.

The guiding rule for radiographic examinations must be the ALARA principle:

Radiation doses to everybody in or in the vicinity of an active X-ray room shall be As Low As Reasonably Achievable (ALARA) taking into account economic and social factors.

That rule will be kept if you follow what is said above in the general principles, and if you follow the instructions for examinations given in this manual.

And always remember:

X-RAYS MAY CAUSE HARM EVEN IF YOU DO NOT SEE OR FEEL THEM!

How to use the manual

The instructions in the present manual are meant to be self-explanatory. Each page displays one examination. Read through the text, look at the images, and follow the instructions given, step by step.

Techniques: BASIC or ADDITIONAL

All **BASIC** views must be taken whenever an examination is ordered.

ADDITIONAL views are taken only when:

(a) the condition of the patient does not permit a basic view; or

(b) the diagnostic information provided by the basic view is insufficient.

Position of the patient

ERECT	standing or sitting up,
SUPINE	lying on the back,
PRONE	lying on the stomach,
DECUBITUS	lying on the side,
OBLIQUE	turned a little, usually at a given angle,
LATERAL	standing or sitting or lying with one side close to the cassette or cassette holder.

X-ray beam direction: AP or PA

AP = Antero–Posterior (front to back) and
PA = Posterior–Anterior (back to front)
indicates the direction of the X-ray beam through the patient onto the cassette.

Instructions on each page

The position of the X-ray equipment.
The cassette size and nominal speed of the screen-film combination (see below).*
When appropriate to use Right or Left marker.
Recommendation to collimate (the X-ray field).
Exposure factors (see below).**
The position of the patient.
An example of resulting radiograph.

* ***Film speed and cassettes***

The speed of the screen-film combination should be written on the cassettes.

In the **"blue" system** (calcium-tungstate and rapid yttrium-tantalate screens) the nominal speed is equal to the actual speed at any kV value. In the manual, the used speeds of the screen-film combinations are 50 and 200 for the "blue" system.

In the **"green" system** (gadolinium-oxysulfide) the actual speed varies with the kV value, low speed at low kV values, nominal speed at 70–75 kV and a little higher speed at higher kV values. In the manual, the used speeds of the screen-film combinations are 100, 200, and 400 for the "green" system. Actual speed is shown for different kV values as nominal speed/actual speed, for example 100/63 and 400/500.

In a few cases a loose grid is recommended, but a grid cassette is preferable.

** ***Exposure factors***

The presented exposure values are based on a standard **WHIS-RAD installation**, with a focus-film distance (FFD) of 140 cm, a fixed Pb/Al grid (with a ratio of 10:1 and 40 lines/cm focused at 135–140 cm) built into the cassette holder. Where shown, the cassette is placed outside the cassette holder, adjacent to the body part examined.

The exposure factors are based on a **"reference man"** with a height of 180 cm (6 feet) and a weight of 80 kg (175 lbs).

Note that the exposure factors also are dependent on the brand of screens, brand of films, and the film processing. The values have to be locally adjusted.

Exposure factors for **children** are very difficult to give, depending on the different shape of children with the same weight or age. Approximate values are given but have to be individually adjusted.

The **kV** value will determine the contrast in the image.

The **mAs** value will determine the image blackening.

For **detailed exposure tables**, see chapter 11.

Chest

LUNGS AND HEART

Patients able to stand

1. Chest PA, page 6.
2. Chest lateral, page 7.

Patients unable to stand but able to sit

3. Chest AP, page 8.
4. Chest lateral, page 9.

Patients lying down, unable to stand or sit

5. Chest AP, page 10.

Other additional views

6. Chest apical (lordotic) AP, page 11.
7. Chest lateral decubitus AP or PA, page 12.

RIBS

A Chest PA 1, or a Chest AP 3, or a Chest AP 5, as described above must always be taken first.

Patients able to either stand or sit

8. Ribs oblique AP, page 13.
   Two views to be taken

Patients lying down, unable to stand or sit

9. Ribs oblique AP, page 14.

INFANTS WEIGHING UP TO 10–15 kg – LUNGS AND HEART

10. Chest AP erect, page 15.
11. Chest AP supine, page 16.

CHEST PA Standing erect BASIC

Cassette speed
Cassette with screen-film combination, nominal speed 200 in the cassette holder

Cassette size
35×43 cm (14×17 inches)
35×35 cm (14×14 inches)
24×30 cm (10×12 inches) for a child
Use a **R**ight or **L**eft marker

Exposure values	kV	mAs average	mAs range
Adult	120	2–2.5	1–12
Child	90	1.6–2	1–4

1. Bring in the patient, decide the cassette format and put the cassette in the cassette holder. Collimate to that format.
2. Position the patient, make sure the patient's shoulders are well pressed forward. Collimate further, if possible.
3. Tell the patient to take a deep breath and hold the breath in.
4. Expose.
5. Tell the patient to breathe normally.

For INFANTS weighing less than 10 and SMALL CHILDREN 15 kg, see CHEST 10 or CHEST 11.

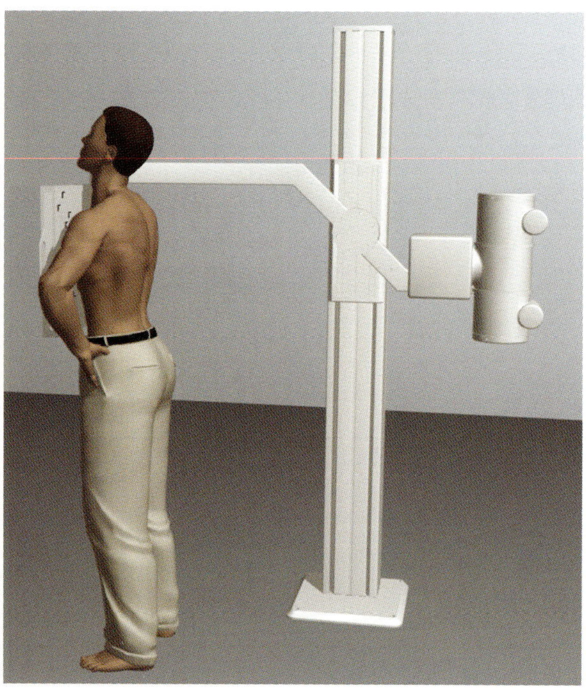

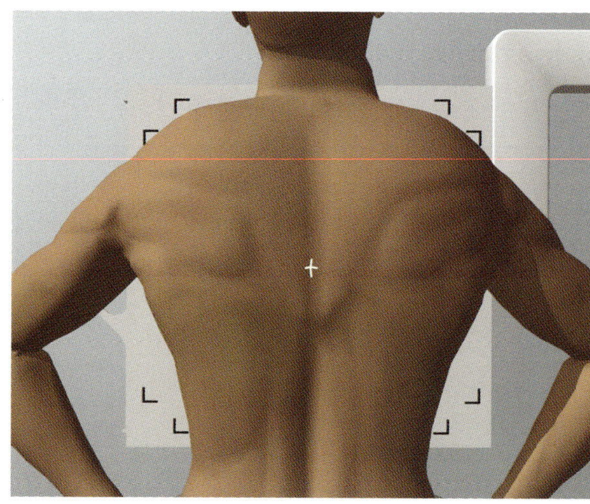

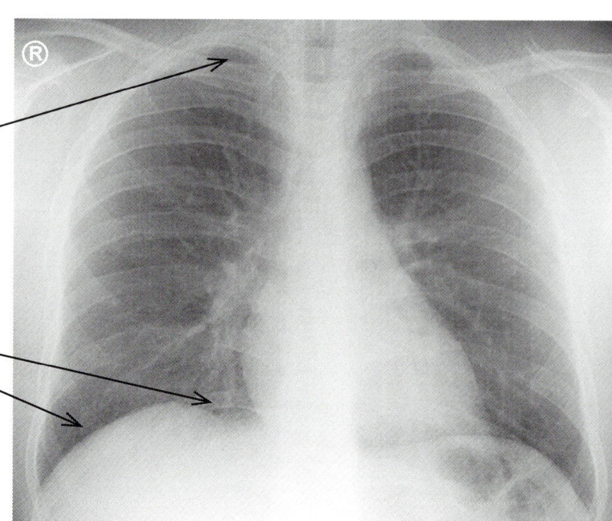

Comments

The top of the lungs must be visible.

The exposure shall be made at full inspiration: rib 10 shall be visible posteriorly above the diaphragm and rib 6 anteriorly.

Make sure that the lower parts of the diaphragm is visible on both sides, including both costophrenic angles.

The lung structure and the spine must be discernible (seen) behind the heart.

CHEST LATERAL Standing erect – left (or right) BASIC

Cassette speed
Cassette with screen-film combination, nominal speed 200 in the cassette holder

Cassette size
35×43 cm (14×17 inches)
35×35 cm (14×14 inches)
24×30 cm (10×12 inches) for a child

Exposure values	kV	mAs average	mAs range
Adult	120	4–5	2–16
Child	90	2.5	1–5

1. Bring in the patient, decide the cassette format and put the cassette in the cassette holder. Collimate to that format.
2. Position the patient,(normally left lateral as shown). The patient should be upright or leaning slightly forwards, not backwards. Use the cassette holder arm for support. Collimate further, if possible.
3. Tell the patient to take a deep breath and hold the breath in.
4. Expose.
5. Tell the patient to breathe normally.

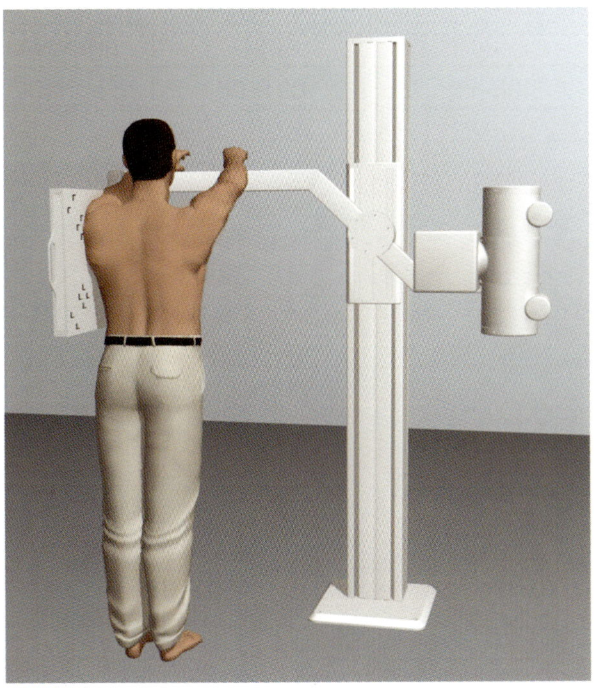

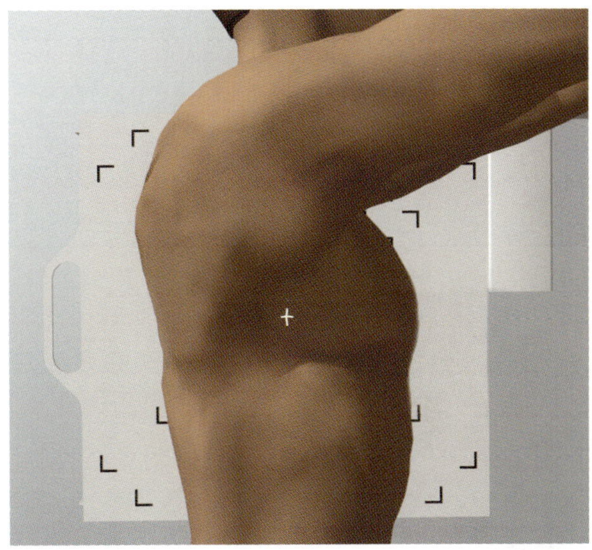

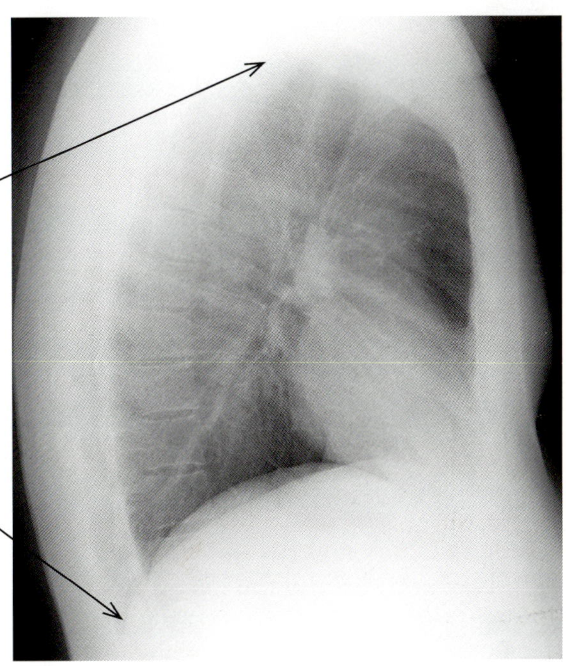

Comments

The top of the lungs must be visible.

Straight lateral view of the sternum

Make sure that the lower parts of the diaphragm is visible.

CHEST AP Sitting erect

on a stool or trolley – only used when the patient is unable to stand

Cassette speed
Cassette with screen-film combination, nominal speed 200 in the cassette holder

Cassette size
35×43 cm (14×17 inches)
35×35 cm (14×14 inches)
24×30 cm (10×12 inches) for a child
Use a **R**ight or **L**eft marker

Exposure values	kV	mAs average	mAs range
Adult	120	2–2.5	1–12
Child	90	1.6–2	1–4

1. Bring in the patient, decide the cassette format and put the cassette in the cassette holder. Collimate to that format.
2. Position the patient, make sure the patient is sitting erect! Collimate further, if possible.
3. Tell the patient to take a deep breath and hold the breath in.
4. Expose.
5. Tell the patient to breathe normally.

For INFANTS weighing less than 10 and SMALL CHILDREN 15 kg, see CHEST 10 or CHEST 11.

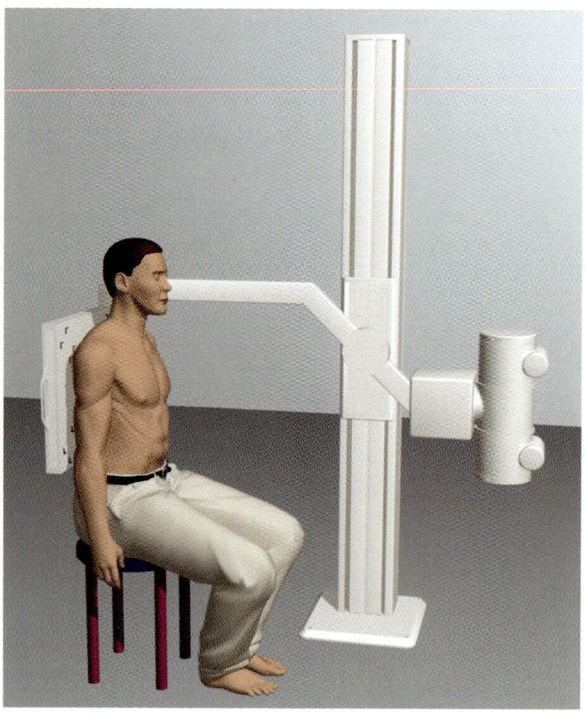

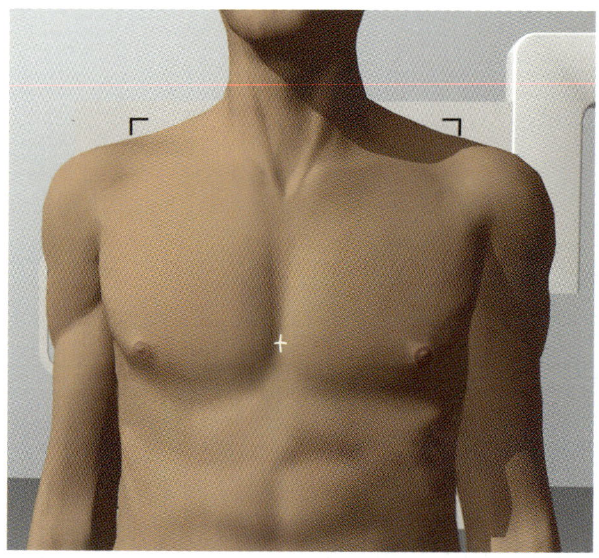

Comments

The top of the lungs must be visible.

The exposure shall be made at full inspiration.

Make sure that the lower parts of the diaphragm is visible on both sides, including both costophrenic angles.

The lung structure and the spine must be discernible (seen) behind the heart.

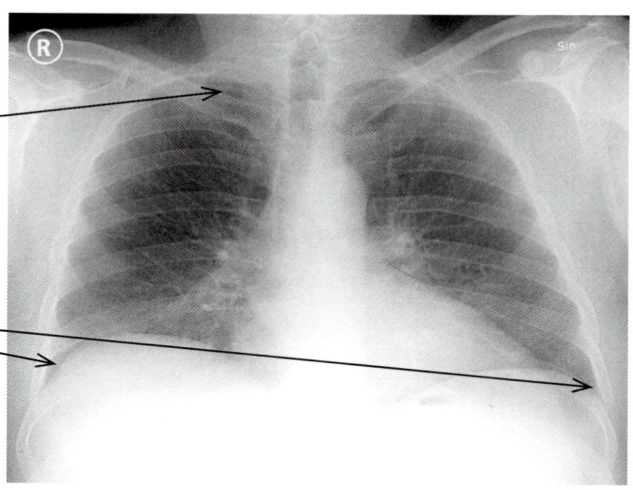

CHEST LATERAL Sitting erect – left (or right) on a stool or trolley – only used when the patient is unable to stand

Cassette speed
Cassette with screen-film combination, nominal speed 200 in the cassette holder

Cassette size
35×43 cm (14×17 inches)
35×35 cm (14×14 inches)
24×30 cm (10×12 inches) for a child

Exposure values	kV	mAs average	mAs range
Adult	120	4–5	2–16
Child	90	2.5	1–5

1. Bring in the patient, decide the cassette format and put the cassette in the cassette holder. Collimate to that format.
2. Position the patient. The patient should be upright or leaning slightly forwards, not backwards. Use the cassette holder arm for support. Collimate further, if possible.
3. Tell the patient to take a deep breath and hold the breath in.
4. Expose.
5. Tell the patient to breathe normally.

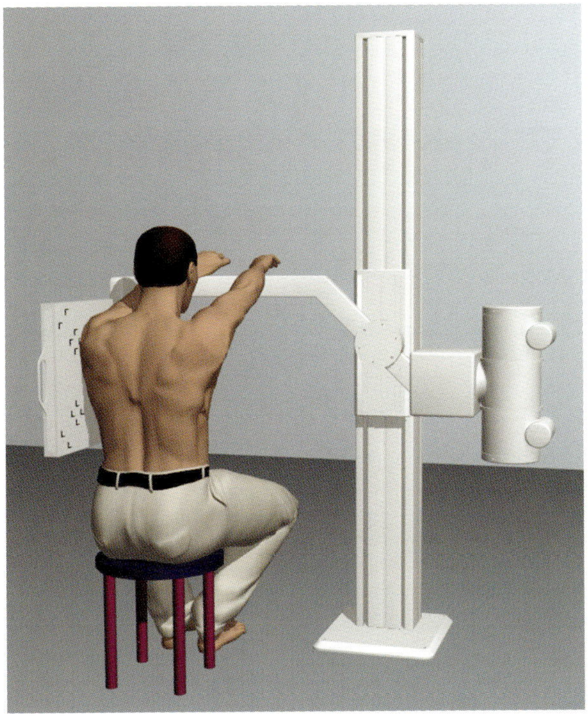

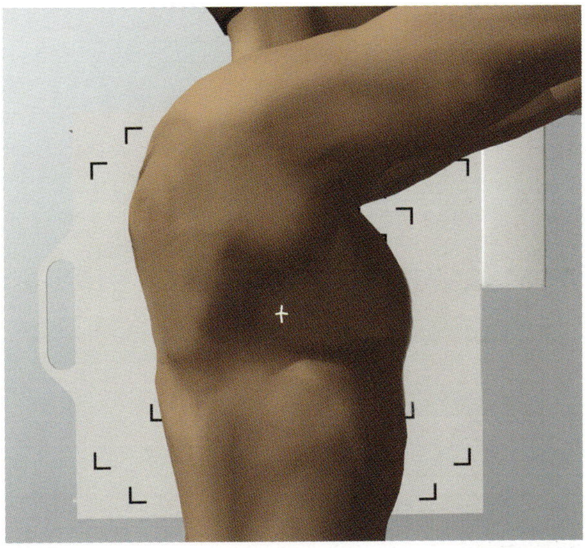

Comments

The top of the lungs must be visible.

Straight lateral view of the sternum

Make sure that the lower parts of the diaphragm is visible.

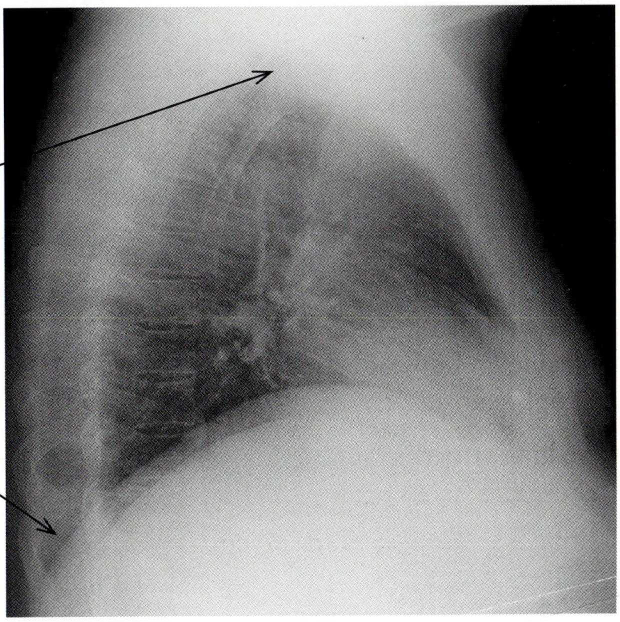

CHEST AP Supine

Cassette speed
Cassette with screen-film combination, nominal speed 200 in the cassette holder

Cassette size
35×43 cm (14×17 inches)
35×35 cm (14×14 inches)
24×30 cm (10×12 inches) for a child
Use a **R**ight or **L**eft marker

Exposure values	kV	mAs average	mAs range
Adult	120	2–3.2	1–12
Child	90	1.6–2	1–4

1. Bring in the patient, decide the cassette format and put the cassette in the cassette holder. Collimate to that format.
2. Position the patient. Put a small pillow under the head. Centre. Collimate further, if possible.
3. Tell the patient to take a deep breath and hold the breath in.
4. Expose.
5. Tell the patient to breathe normally.

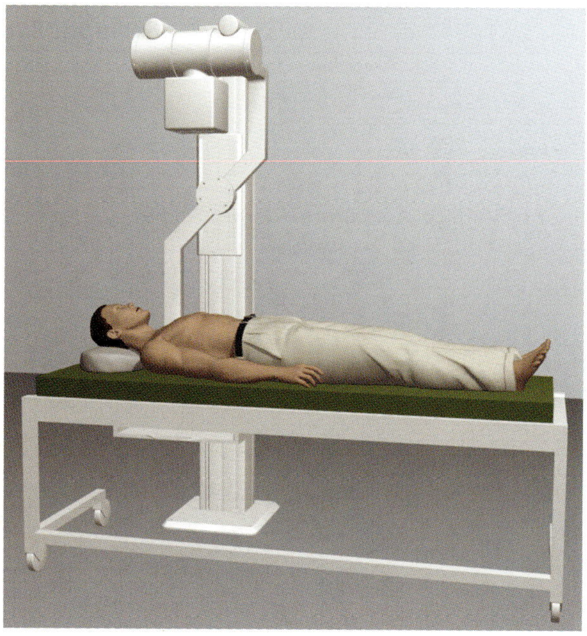

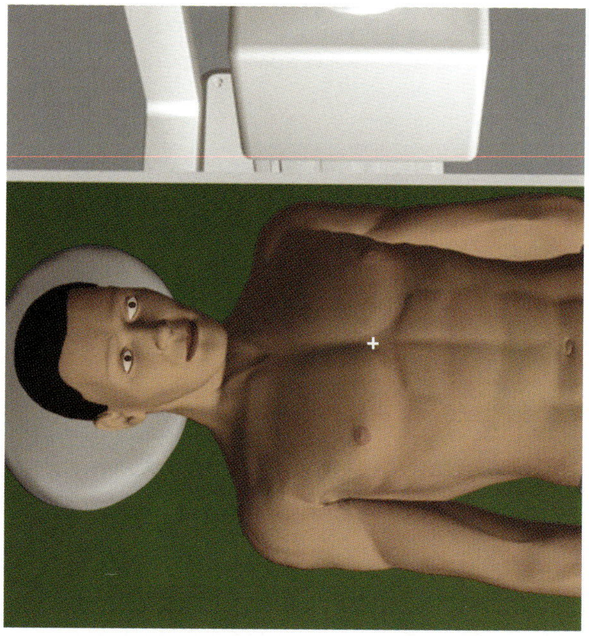

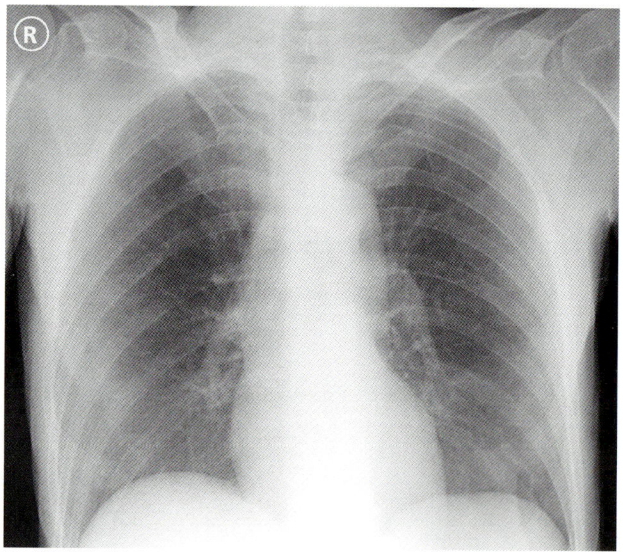

Comments

The top of the lungs must be visible.

The exposure shall be made at full inspiration.

Make sure that the lower parts of the diaphragm is visible on both sides, including both costophrenic angles.

The lung structure and the spine must be discernible (seen) behind the heart.

CHEST APICAL (LORDOTIC) AP Sitting reclining backwards ADDITIONAL

Cassette speed
Cassette with screen-film combination, nominal speed 200 in the cassette holder

Cassette size
24×30 cm (10×12 inches)
Use a **R**ight or **L**eft marker

Exposure values	kV	mAs average	mAs range
Adult	120	2.5	2–5

1. Bring in the patient, put the cassette in the cassette holder. Collimate to the format.
2. Position the patient as shown. Centre.
3. Tell the patient to take a deep breath and hold the breath in.
4. Expose.
5. Tell the patient to breathe normally.

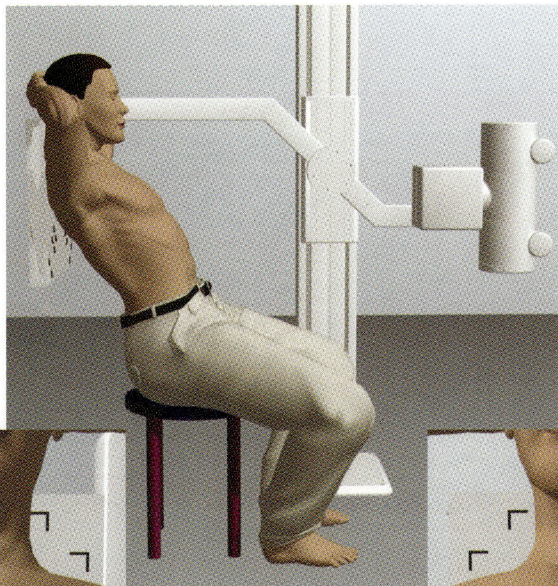

Right side

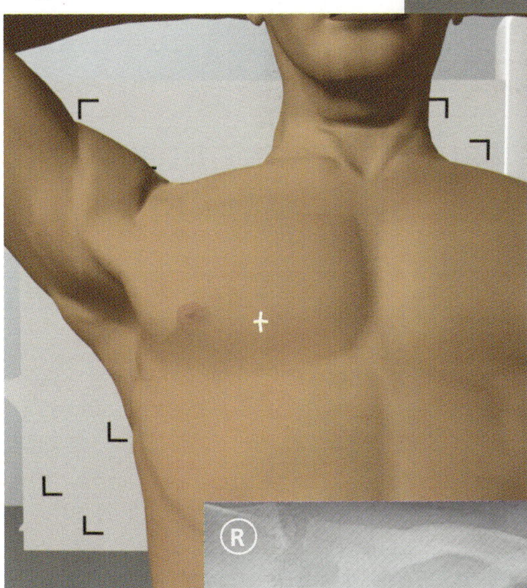

Left side

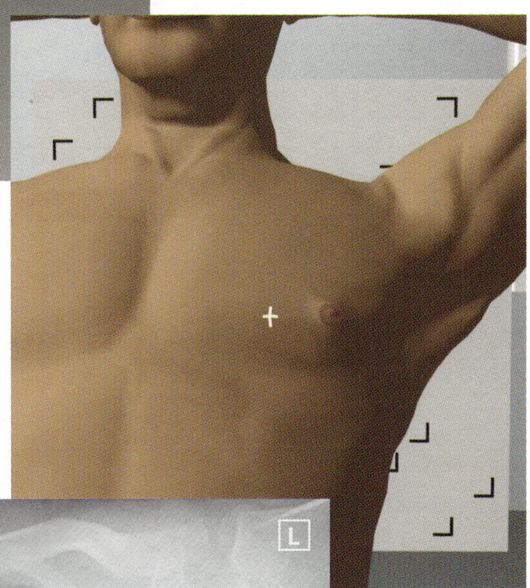

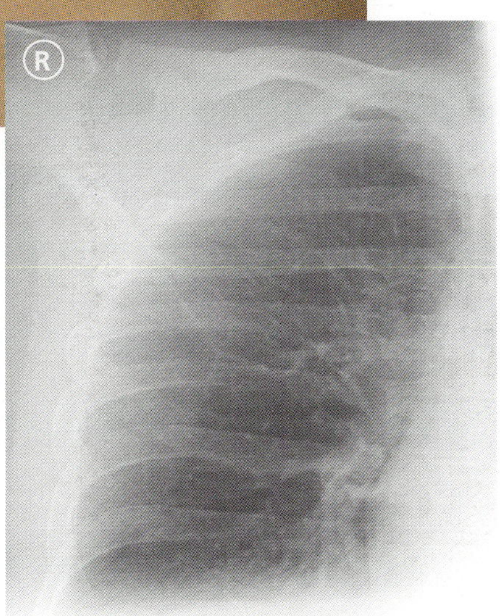

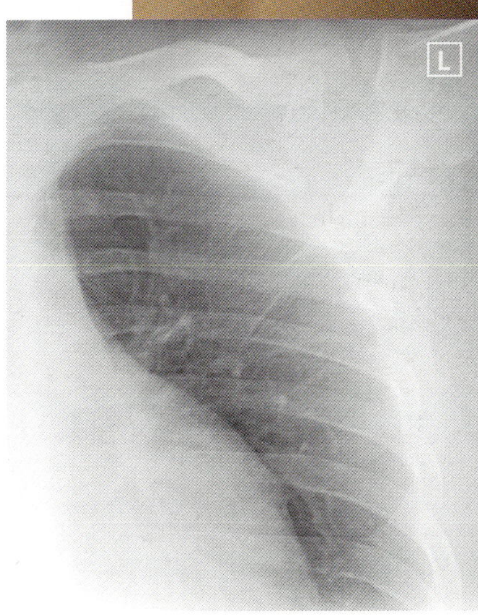

CHEST LATERAL DECUBITUS Lying on the right (PA) or left (AP) side – horizontal beam

ADDITIONAL views used to detect fluid in the pleural sac

Cassette speed
Cassette with screen-film combination, nominal speed 200 in the cassette holder

Cassette size
24×30 cm (10×12 inches)
Use a **R**ight or **L**eft marker

Exposure values	kV	mAs average	mAs range
Adult	120	2	1.6–3.2

1. Bring in the patient, put the cassette in the cassette holder. Collimate to the format.
2. Position the patient, as shown. The patient must lie on the side where the fluid is suspected, close to the cassette holder on 2 hard pillows (with a distance). Centre.
3. Tell the patient to breathe OUT and hold the breath OUT.
4. Expose.
5. Tell the patient to breathe normally.

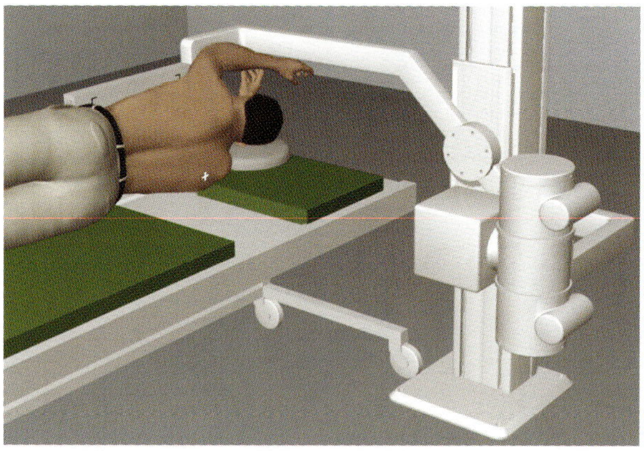

Position for RIGHT lateral decubitus

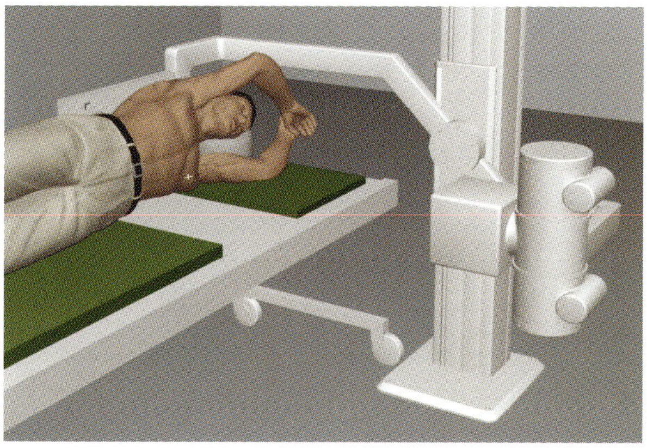

Position for LEFT lateral decubitus

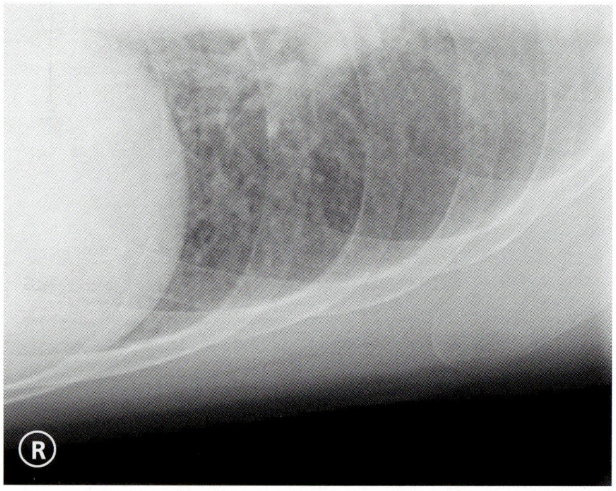

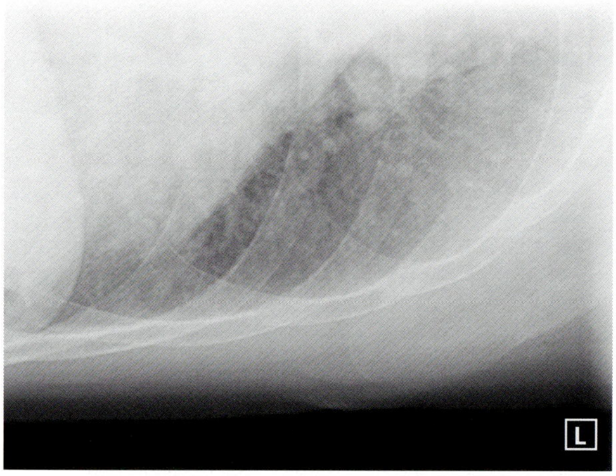

RIBS OBLIQUE AP Standing or sitting erect – right and left oblique BASIC

CHEST 1 or CHEST 3 or CHEST 5 must always be taken first

Cassette speed
Cassette with screen-film combination, nominal speed 200 in the cassette holder

Cassette size
35×43 cm (14×17 inches)
35×35 cm (14×14 inches)
Use a **R**ight or **L**eft marker

Exposure values	kV	mAs average	mAs range
Adult	70	20–25	10–125

1. Bring in the patient, put the cassette in the cassette holder. Collimate to the format.
2. Position the patient as shown. IF THE PATIENT IS UNABLE TO RAISE HIS ARMS, THE ARMS SHOULD BE HELD OUT FROM THE BODY. Collimate further, if possible. Centre.
3. Tell the patient to take a deep breath and hold the breath in.
4. Expose.
5. Tell the patient to breathe normally.

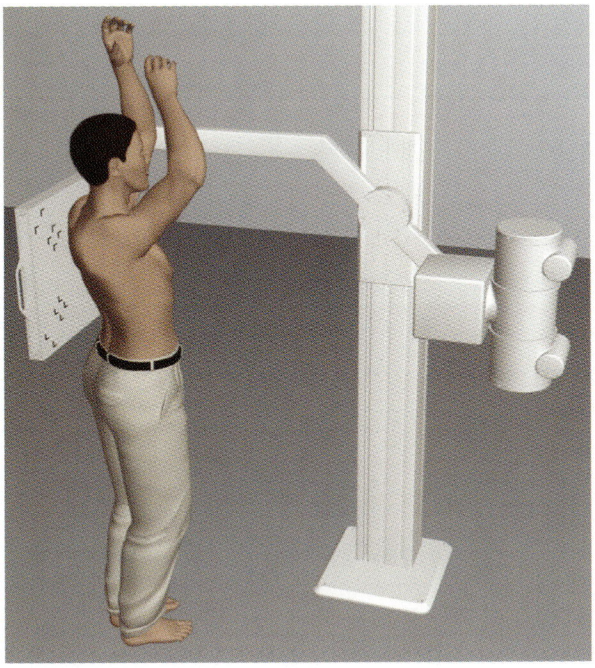

Left oblique

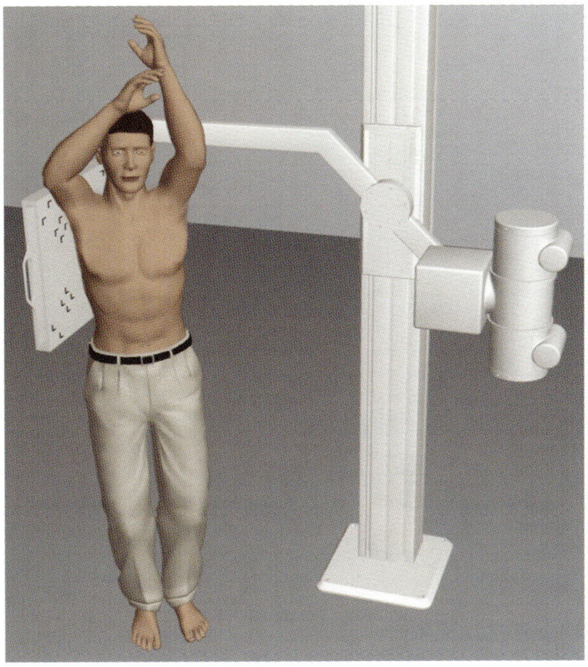

Right oblique

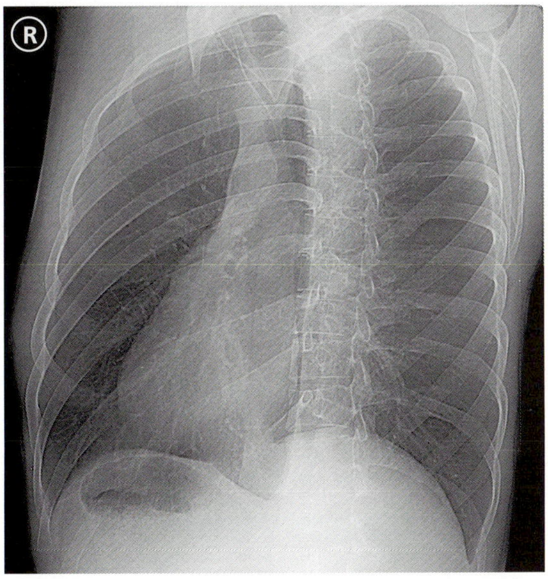

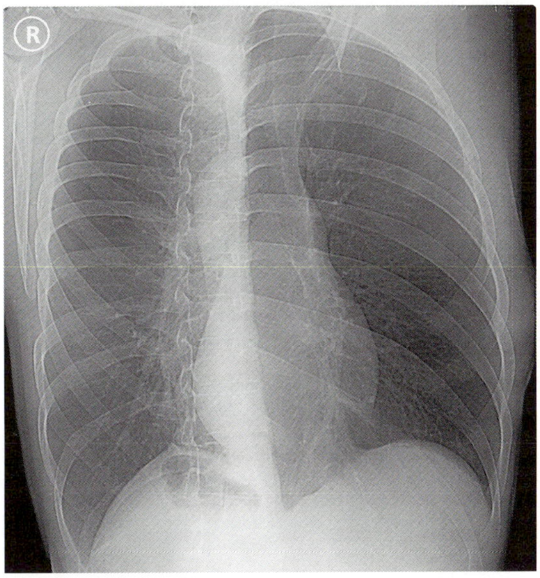

RIBS OBLIQUE AP Supine – right and left oblique

CHEST 1 or CHEST 3 or CHEST 5 must always be taken first

Cassette speed
Cassette with screen-film combination, nominal speed 200 in the cassette holder

Cassette size
35×43 cm (14×17 inches)
35×35 cm (14×14 inches)
Use a **R**ight or **L**eft marker

Exposure values	kV	mAs average	mAs range
Adult	70	20–25	10–125

1. Bring in the patient, put the cassette in the cassette holder. Collimate to the format.
2. Position the patient as shown. SUPPORT THE PATIENT WITH A PILLOW UNDER THE NORMAL SIDE. Keep the UPPER arm as high as possible. Collimate further, if possible. Centre.
3. Tell the patient to take a deep breath and hold the breath in.
4. Expose.
5. Tell the patient to breathe normally.

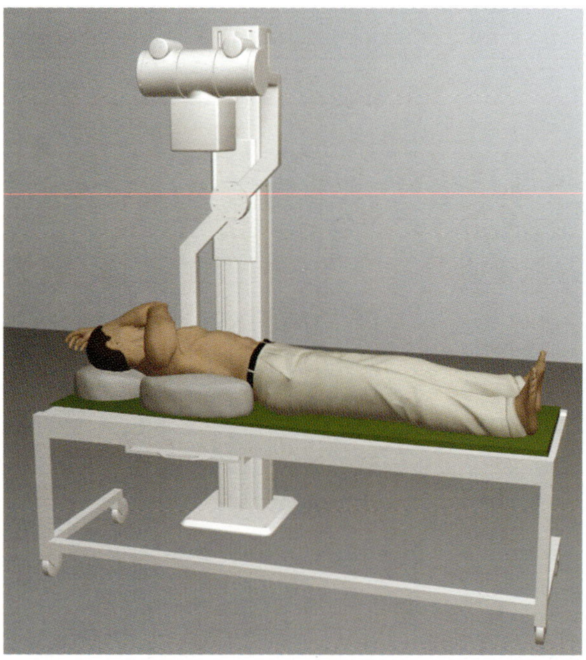

Left oblique

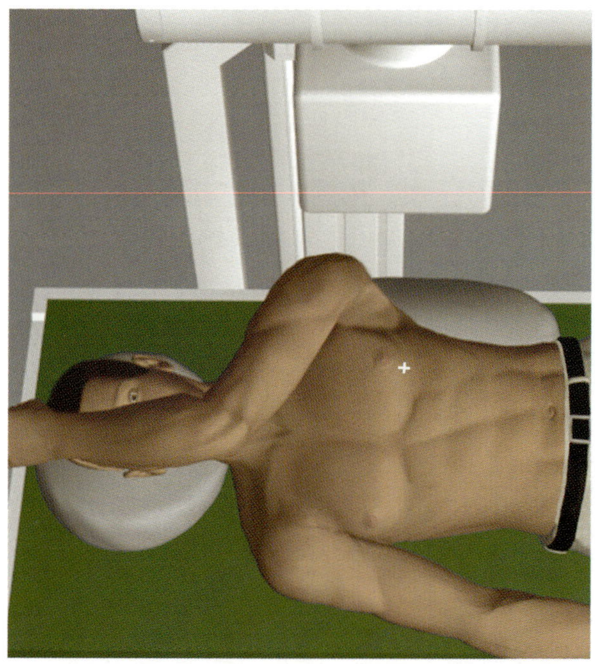

Right oblique

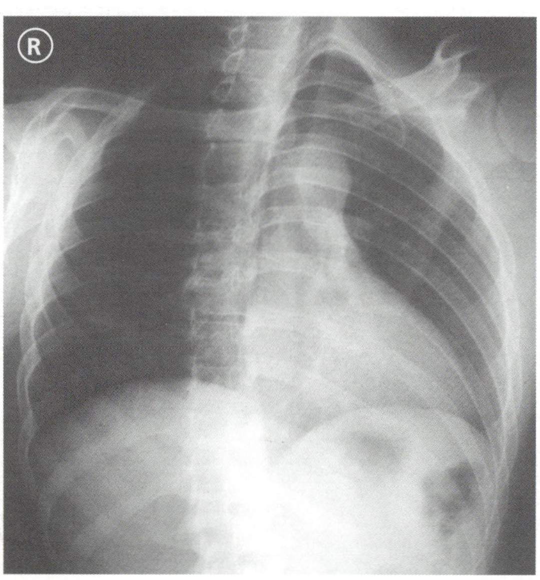

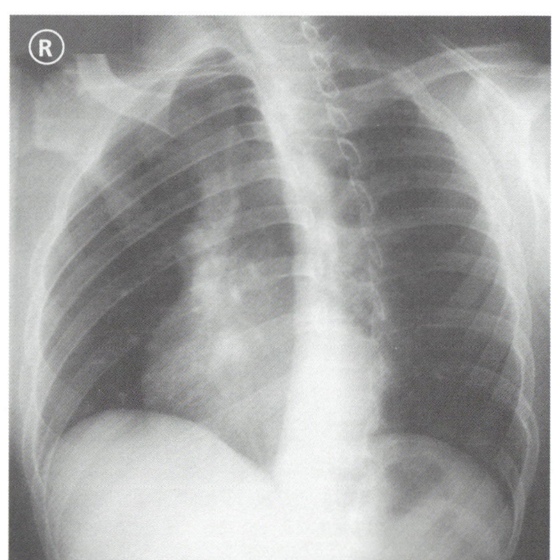

CHEST AP Erect BASIC

Infants and small children weighing up to 15 kg, hanging by the upper arms

Cassette speed
Cassette with screen-film combination, nominal speed 200 **in** the cassette holder

Cassette size
24×30 cm (10×12 inches)
Use a **R**ight or **L**eft marker

Exposure values	kV	mAs range
Child	90	1.25–2.5

1. Bring in the patient, put the cassette in the cassette holder. Collimate to the format.
2. Position the patient. The child is held hanging by the upper arms (if possible, its feet can be supported by a stool or the floor or by another person holding the thighs) with its back resting against the front of the cassette holder.
3. THE PERSON(S) HOLDING THE CHILD, preferably one of the parents, MUST WEAR A LEAD APRON and, whenever possible, LEAD GLOVES.
4. Centre between the nipples. Collimate further, if possible.
5. Expose when the infant is not moving, preferably in INSPIRATION.

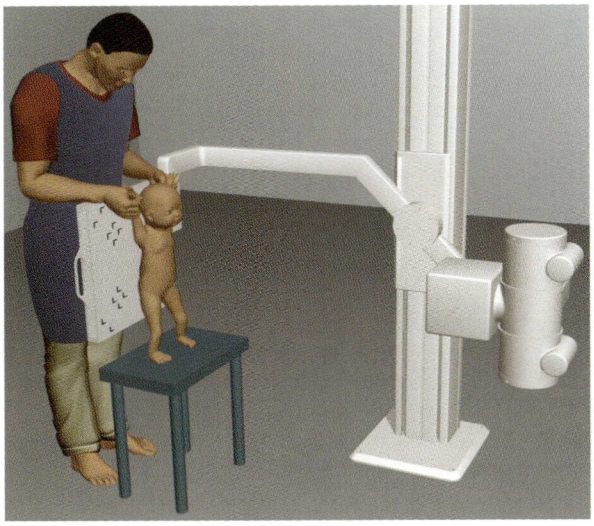

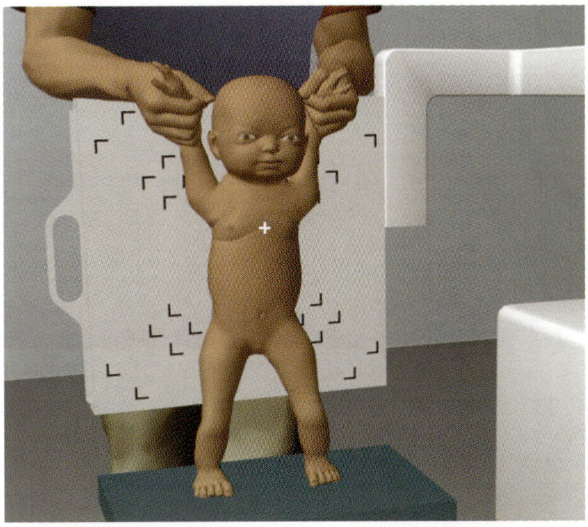

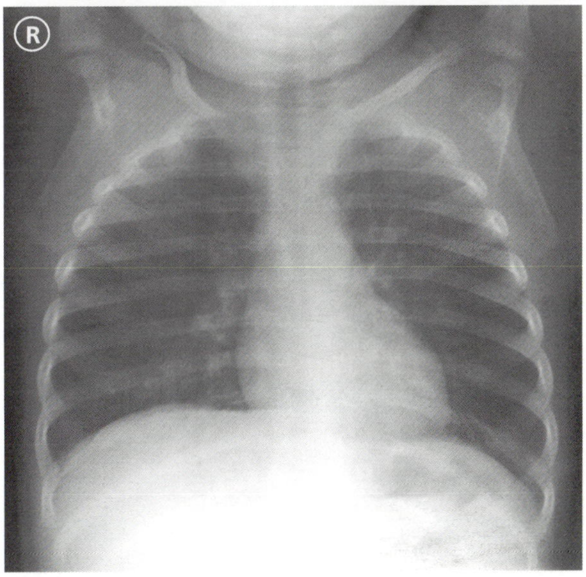

Comment

The person holding the child must wear a lead apron, and, whenever possible, lead gloves.

CHEST AP – infant weighing up to 10 kg   Supine

Cassette speed
Cassette with screen-film combination, nominal speed 200 **on** the cassette holder

Cassette size
18×24 cm (8×10 inches)
Use a **R**ight or **L**eft marker

Exposure values	kV	mAs range
Child	70	1.6–3.2

1. Centre the cassette on top of the cassette holder. Collimate to that format.
2. Lie the infant on its back on the cassette. THE INFANTS HEAD AND LEGS MUST BE SUPPORTED. THOSE SUPPORTING, preferably the infant's parents, MUST WEAR LEAD APRONS, and, whenever possible, LEAD GLOVES.
3. Centre between the nipples. Collimate further, if possible.
4. Expose when the infant is not moving, preferably in INSPIRATION.

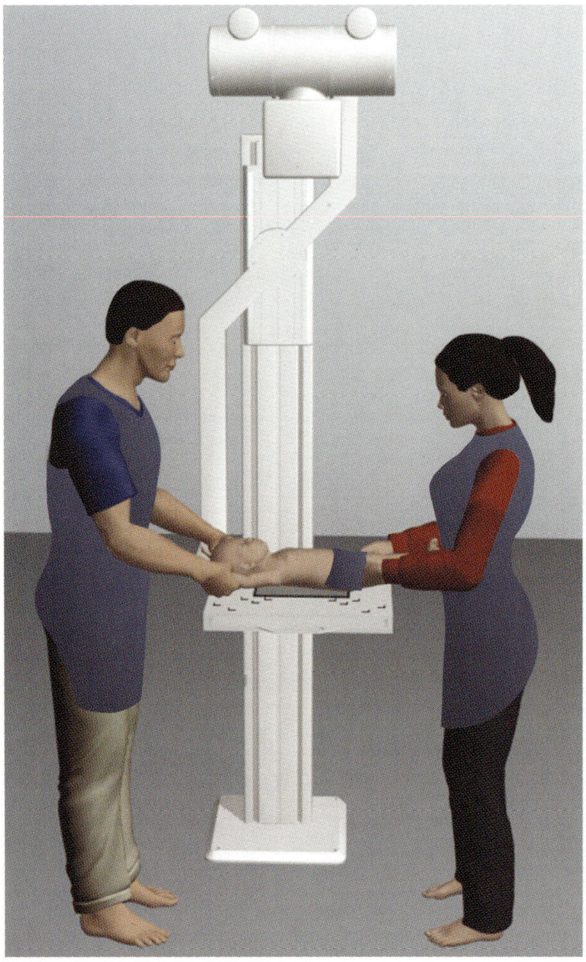

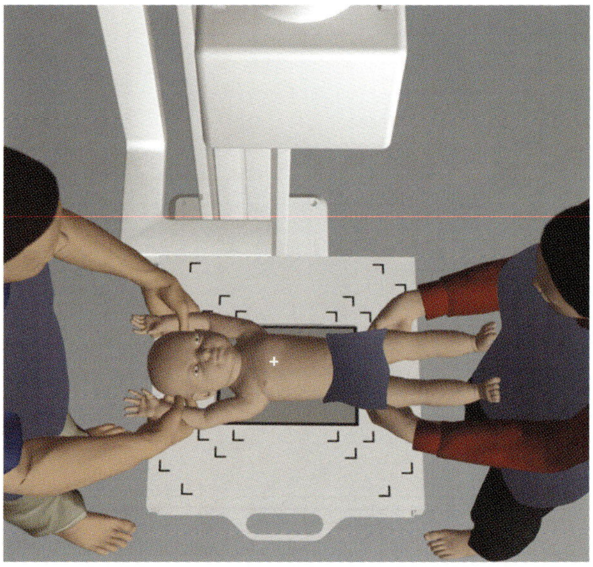

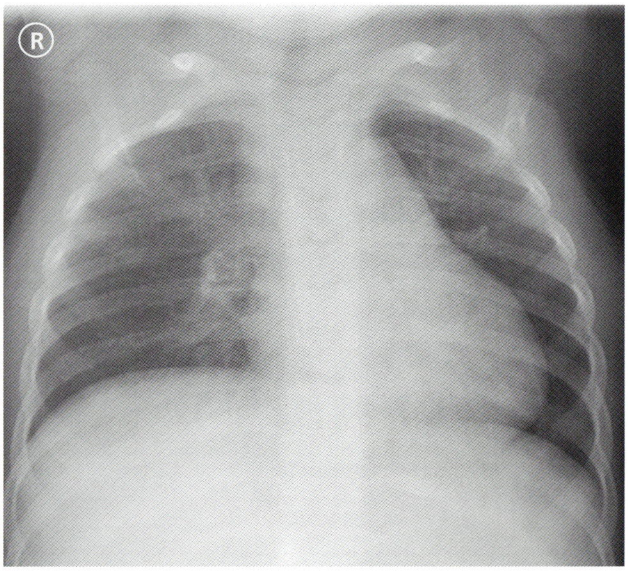

Comments

The persons holding the child must wear lead aprons and, whenever possible, lead gloves.

Use a protective lead strip over the infant's pelvic area.

Abdomen

ABDOMEN GENERAL

X-rays of the abdomen are usually taken with the patient lying down; erect views are taken only when the clinical diagnosis is "acute abdomen", e.g., intestinal obstruction or perforation of the gut.

Patient diagnosed as "acute abdomen", able to stand

1. Acute abdomen AP supine, page 18.
2. Acute abdomen AP standing erect, page 19.

Patient diagnosed as "acute abdomen", unable to stand

Acute abdomen AP supine (see ABDOMEN 1).

3. Acute abdomen lateral decubitus, page 20.
   Two views have to be taken.

Non acute abdomen

Use ABDOMEN 1 (page 18) or ABDOMEN 5 (page 22).

INFANTS AND SMALL CHILDREN WEIGHING UP TO 15 kg

Acute abdomen AP supine (see ABDOMEN 1, page 18).

4. Abdomen AP (hanging), page 21.

URINARY TRACT

X-rays of the urinary tract are taken with the patient lying down.

5. Urinary tract survey AP, page 22.
6. Urinary bladder and inner pelvis, page 23.
7. Intravenous urography, pages 24–29.
   Follow the stepwise instructions (ABDOMEN 7.1–7.4, pages 26–29).

PREGNANCY

When obstructed labour (disproportion) is suspected
NOT TO BE TAKEN BEFORE THE 37th WEEK OF PREGNANCY

8. Pregnancy lateral erect, page 30.

To view the position of the fetus
NOT TO BE TAKEN BEFORE THE 37th WEEK OF PREGNANCY

9. Pregnancy PA, page 31.

ABDOMEN AP Supine BASIC

Cassette speed
Cassette with screen-film combination, nominal speed 200/400 in the cassette holder

Cassette size
35×43 cm (14×17 inches)
24×30 cm (10×12 inches) for a child
Use a **R**ight or **L**eft marker

Exposure values	mAs	
70 **kV**	"blue" system 200	"green" system 400
Average	80	40
Range	50–100	25–50
Child 30 kg	40	20

1. Bring in the patient, decide the cassette format and put the cassette in the cassette holder. Collimate to that format.
2. Position the patient. Put a small pillow under the head. Centre.
   Collimate further, if possible.
3. Tell the patient to breathe OUT and hold the breathe OUT. Expose.
4. Tell the patient to breathe normally.

For INFANTS and SMALL CHILDREN weighing up to 15 kg, see ABDOMEN 4.

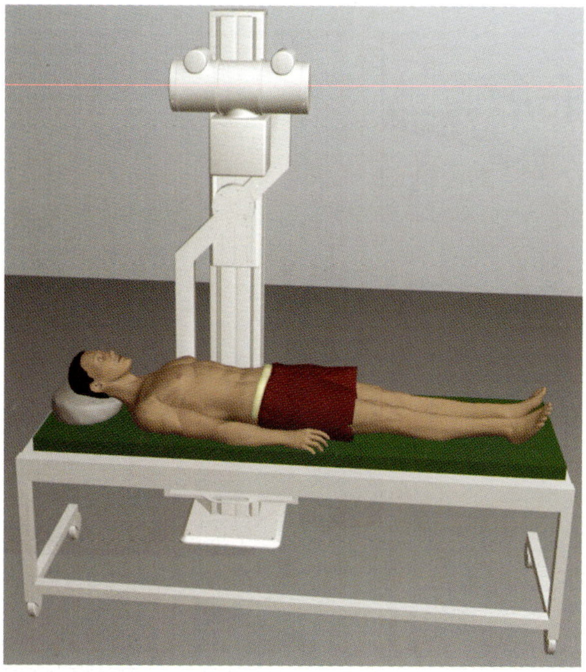

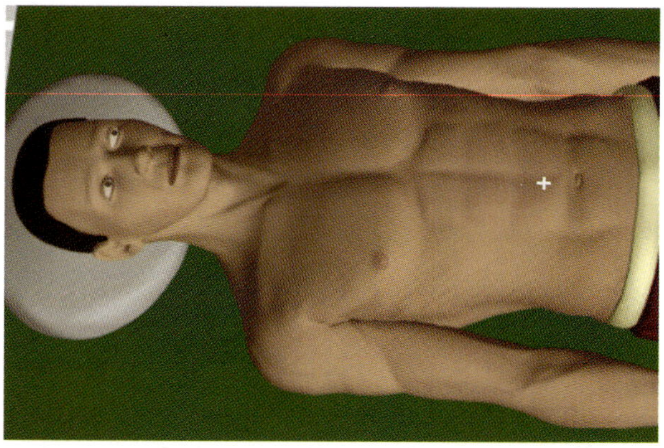

Comments

The diaphragm must be visible; if it is not, change the centre and take a new film.

The pubic symphysis must also be visible; if it is not, take an ABDOMEN 6 (urinary bladder view).

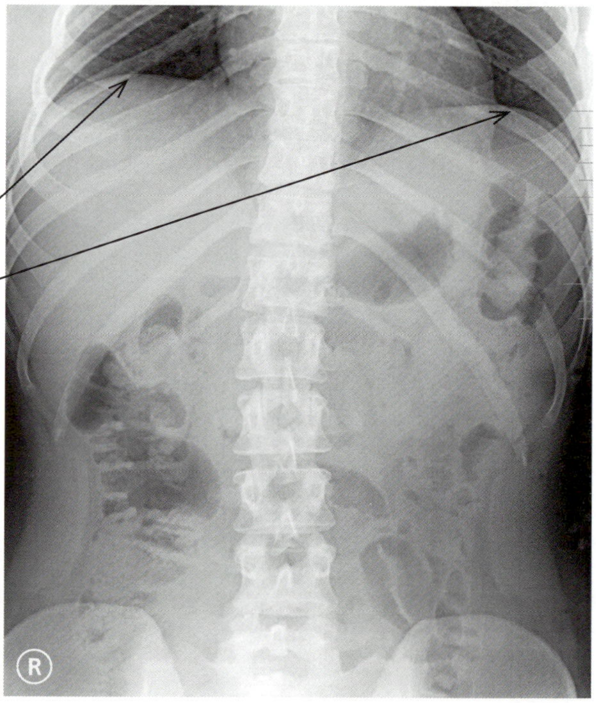

ABDOMEN AP: "ACUTE ABDOMEN" Standing erect BASIC

Cassette speed
Cassette with screen-film combination, nominal speed 200/400 in the cassette holder

Cassette size
35×43 cm (14×17 inches)
24×30 cm (10×12 inches) for a child
Use a **R**ight or **L**eft marker

Exposure values	mAs	
80 kV	"blue" system 200	"green" system 400/450
Average	80	25
Range	50–160	16–50
Child 30 kg	32	12.5

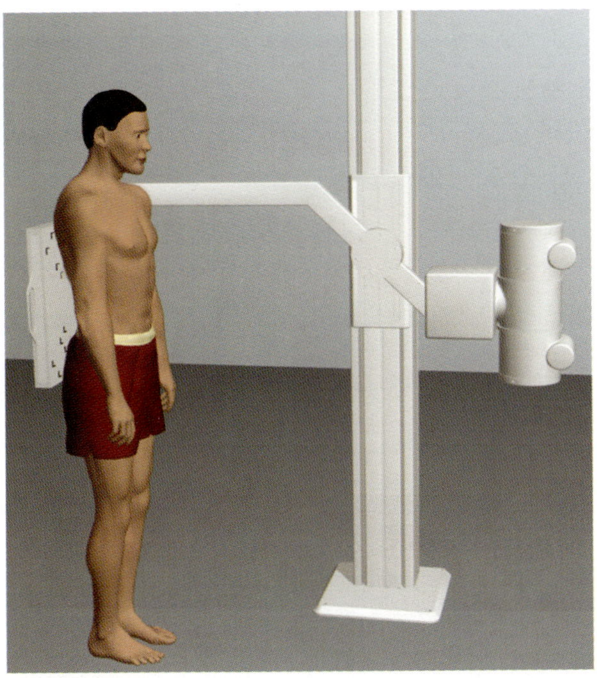

Comments

The diaphragm must be visible; if it is not, change the centre and take a new film.

1. Bring in the patient, decide the cassette format and put the cassette in the cassette holder. Collimate to that format.
2. Position the patient. Press the patient's abdomen against the cassette holder. Centre. Collimate further, if possible.
3. Tell the patient to stop breathing. Expose.
4. Tell the patient to breathe normally.

For INFANTS and SMALL CHILDREN weighing up to 15 kg, see ABDOMEN 4.

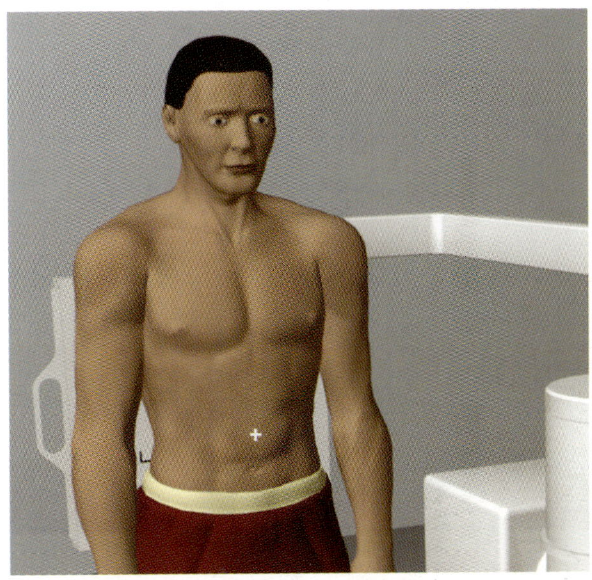

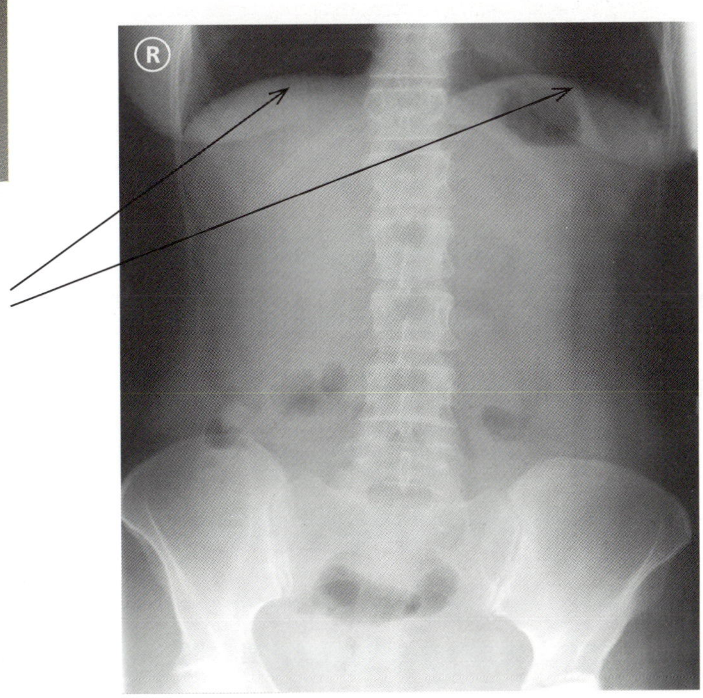

ABDOMEN LATERAL DECUBITUS **Lying first on the left side, then on the right**

Both views to be taken

Cassette speed
Cassette with screen-film combination, nominal speed 200/400 in the cassette holder

Cassette size
35×43 cm (14×17 inches)
Use a **R**ight or **L**eft marker

Exposure values	mAs	
80 kV	"blue" system 200	"green" system 400/450
Average	50	20
Range	40–100	16–40

1. Bring in the patient, put the cassette in the cassette holder. Collimate to the format.
2. Position the patient. THE PATIENT MUST LIE AGAINST THE CASSETTE HOLDER. Centre.
   Collimate further, if possible.
3. Tell the patient to breathe OUT and hold the breath OUT. Expose.
4. Tell the patient to breathe normally.
5. Turn the patient over and repeat.

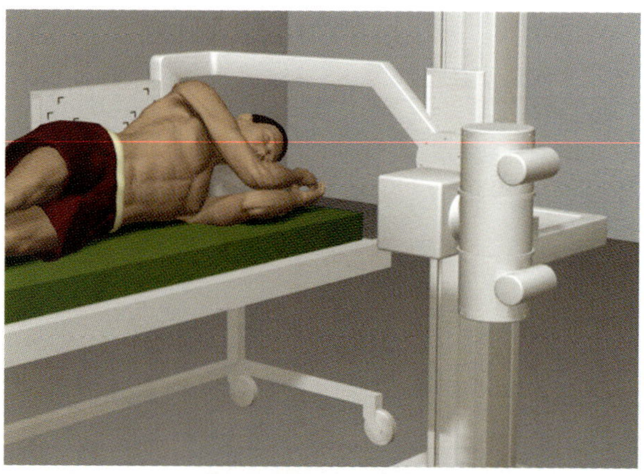

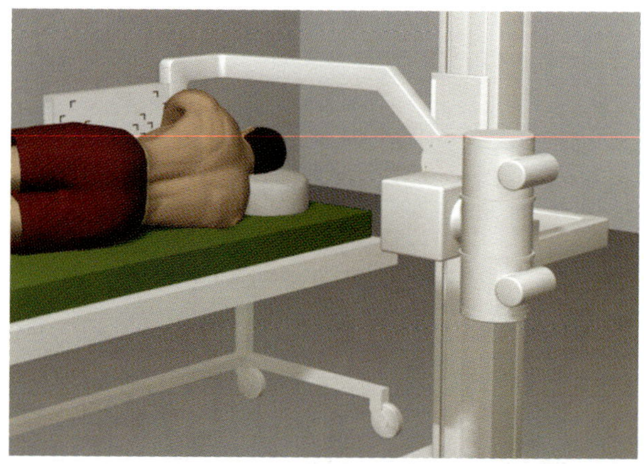

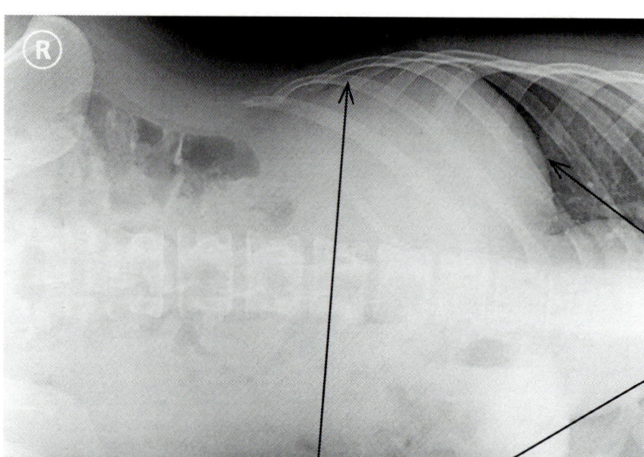

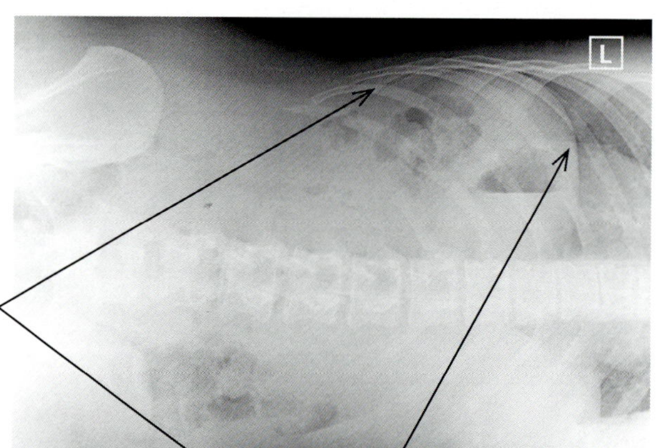

Comments

The upper side of the abdomen must be visible at the top of the films.

The upper part of diaphragm must be visible on the films.

ABDOMEN AP Erect BASIC

Infants and small children weighing up to 15 kg, hanging by the upper arms

Cassette speed

Cassette with screen-film combination, nominal speed 200/400 in the cassette holder

Cassette size

24×30 cm (10×12 inches)

Use a **R**ight or **L**eft marker

Exposure values	mAs	
70 **kV**	"blue" system 200	"green" system 400
Average	20	10
Range	8–32	4–16

1. Bring in the patient, put the cassette in the cassette holder. Collimate to the format.
2. Position the patient. The child is held hanging by the upper arms (if possible, its feet can be supported by a stool or the floor or by another person holding the thighs) with its back resting against the front of the cassette holder.
3. THE PERSON(S) HOLDING THE CHILD, preferably one of the parents, MUST WEAR A LEAD APRON and, whenever possible, LEAD GLOVES.
4. Centre to the navel. Collimate further.
5. Expose when the child is not moving.

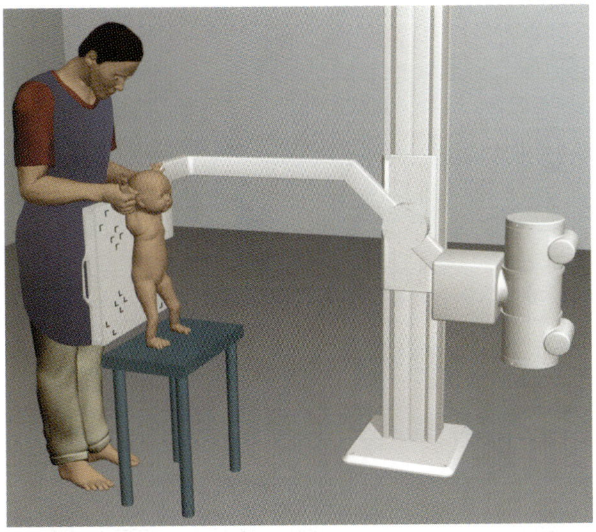

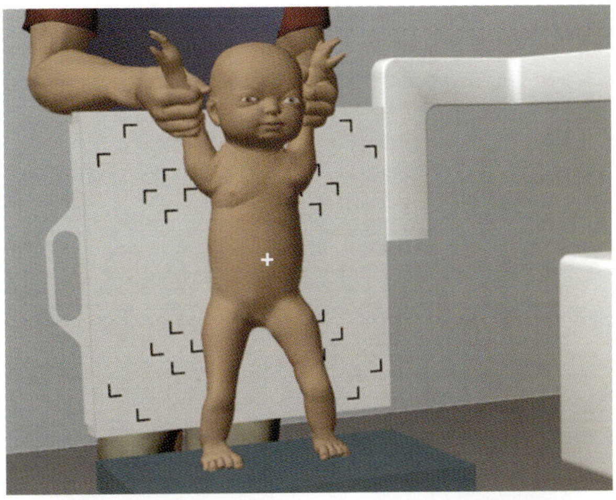

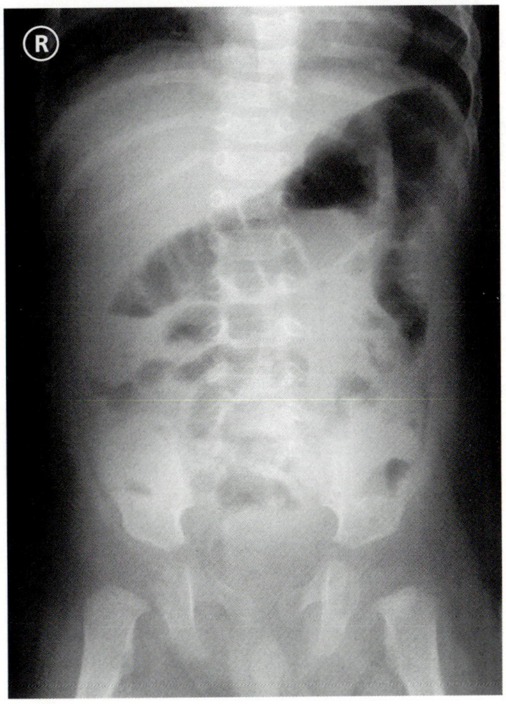

Comments

The person holding the child must wear a lead apron and lead gloves, whenever possible.

The whole abdomen (from diafragm to symfysis) must be included on the film.

URINARY TRACT SURVEY, also NON ACUTE ABDOMEN   Supine   BASIC

Cassette speed
Cassette with screen-film combination, nominal speed 200/400 in the cassette holder

Cassette size
35×43 cm (14×17 inches)
24×30 cm (10×12 inches) for a child
Use a **R**ight or **L**eft marker

Exposure values	mAs (average)	
kV	"blue" system 200	"green" system 400/450
70	125	63
80 with contrast	63	32

1. Bring in the patient, decide the cassette format and put the cassette in the cassette holder. Collimate to that format.
2. Position the patient. Put a small pillow under the head. Centre.
   Collimate further, if possible.
3. Tell the patient to breathe OUT and hold the breath OUT.
4. Expose.
5. Tell the patient to breathe normally.

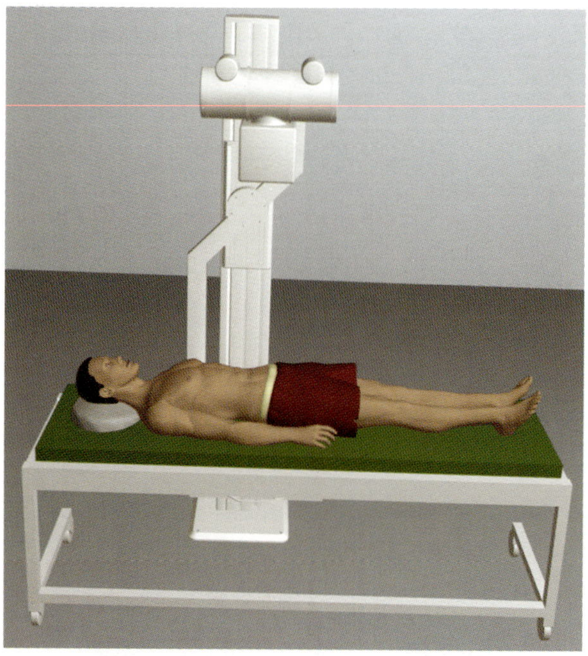

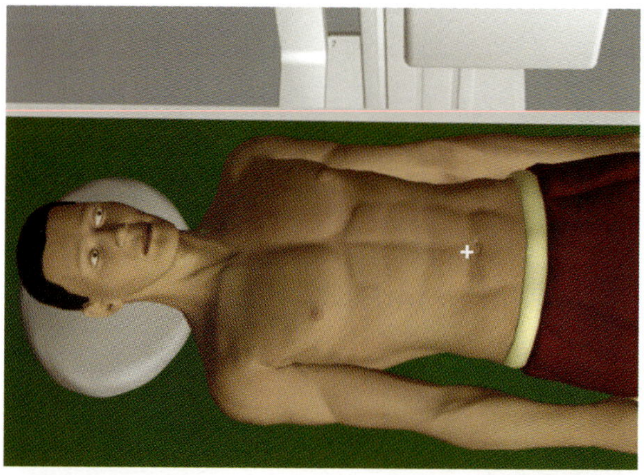

Comments

The lower ribs (the top of the kidneys) must be visible; if it is not, change the centre and take a new film.

The pubic symphysis must be visible; if it is not, take an ABDOMEN 6 (urinary bladder view).

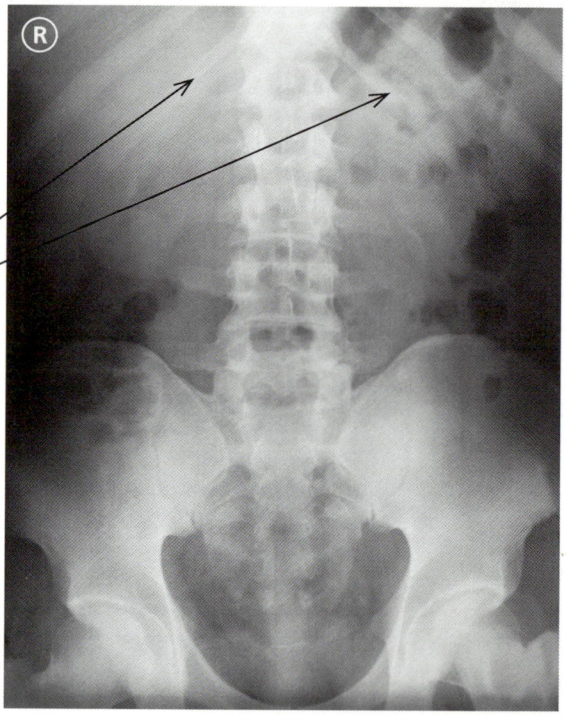

URINARY BLADDER and INNER PELVIS **Supine – vertical beam angled 20° as shown**

BASIC

Cassette speed
Cassette with screen-film combination, nominal speed 200/400 in the cassette holder

Cassette size
24×30 cm (10×12 inches)
Use a **R**ight or **L**eft marker

Exposure values	**mAs** (average)	
kV	"blue" system 200	"green" system 400/450
70	200	100
80 with contrast	100	50

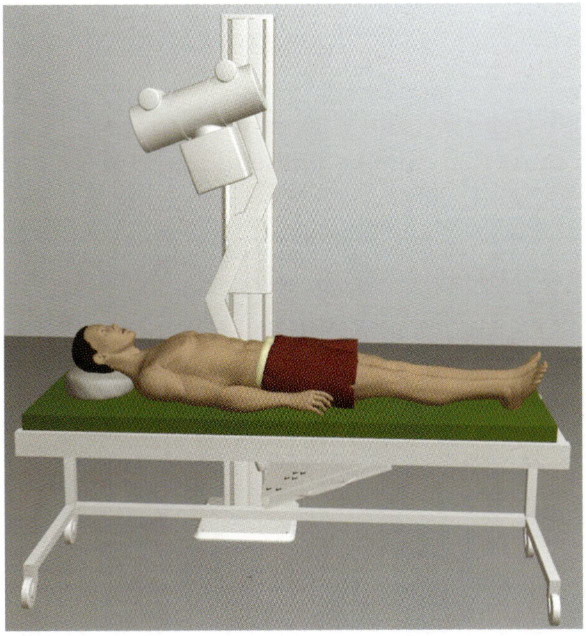

1. Bring in the patient, put the cassette in the cassette holder. Collimate to the format.
2. Position the patient. Put a small pillow under the head. Centre 4 cm above the symphysis. Collimate further, if possible.
3. Tell the patient to hold the breath.
4. Expose.
5. Tell the patient to breathe normally.

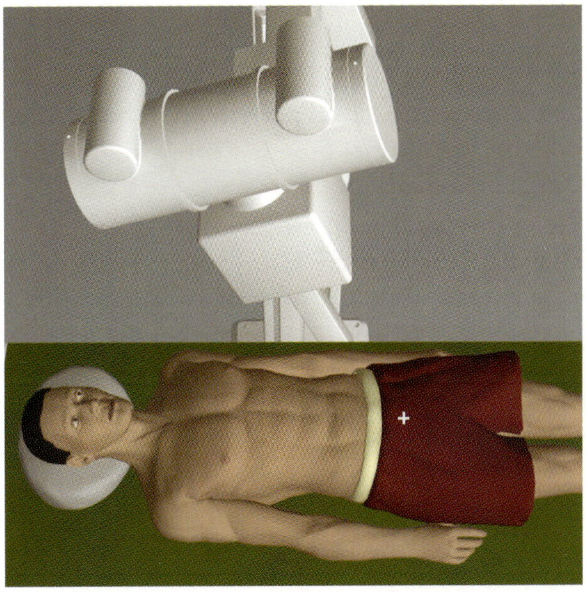

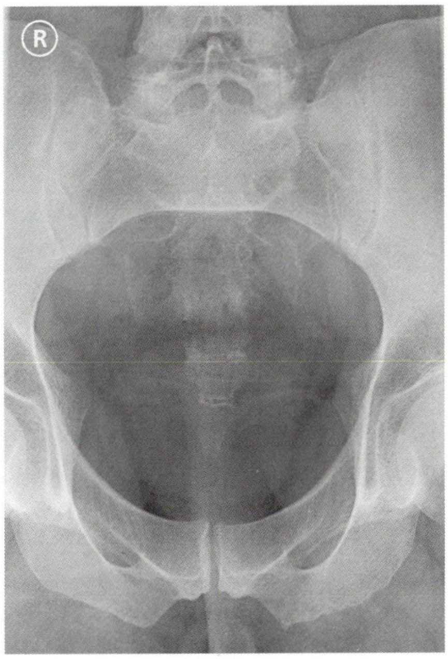

INTRAVENOUS UROGRAPHY:

EXAMINATION OF THE KIDNEYS, URETERS AND BLADDER

OBSERVE: Read this before you go to the procedure (i.e. next page).

The patient will be given an intravenous injection of a contrast medium. Make sure syringe, needles, and contrast medium are ready.

Only media specifically made for intravenous urography should be used. Media for vascular investigations may be too strong and those which are used for filling of the bladder or urethra (cystography, urethrography) may be too weak.

Contrast media come in different concentrations.
Ask the doctor which concentration and which volume to use.

The normal volume (dose) is between 40 ml and 100 ml for adults. For children weighing less than 10 kilogram, 2 ml per kilogram body weight is commonly used, and for children above 10 kilogram the normal dose is 1 ml per kilogram body weight.

Check the contrast medium with the doctor.
A wrong drug may be harmful or even kill the patient.

WARNING: Injection of contrast media may lead to adverse reactions that can be serious. A medical doctor and appropriate drugs for treatment must therefore be immediately available whenever contrast media are given.

Now read the next page which describes the procedure for intravenous urography.

PROCEDURE FOR INTRAVENOUS UROGRAPY

READ THE PREVIOUS PAGE BEFORE YOU START HERE.

ABDOMEN 7.1

1. Ask the patient to empty the bladder or, if there is a catheter in the bladder, open the catheter and drain the urine into a container.
2. Take a urinary tract survey with the patient lying supine (ABDOMEN 5)—FILM 1. FILM 1, page 26
3. If the pelvis is not completely visible on the radiograph adjust the X-ray stand and take a urinary bladder and inner pelvis view (ABDOMEN 6)—FILM 1A. FILM 1A, page 26

ABDOMEN 7.2

4. When FILM 1 (and FILM 1A if taken) have been checked by the DOCTOR, and the X-ray stand has been adjusted if necessary after FILM 1A, the DOCTOR gives the contrast injection.
5. YOU MUST NOTE THE TIME the injection is given.
6. As soon as the injection is given, take a urinary tract survey with the patient lying supine (ABDOMEN 5)—FILM 2. FILM 2, page 27
7. Ten minutes later take another urinary tract survey with the patient lying supine (ABDOMEN 5)—FILM 3. FILM 3, page 27

ABDOMEN 7.3

8. If the doctor confirms that the radiographs are SATISFACTORY, proceed directly to point 11 below. If the kidneys, ureters, and bladder are not sufficiently visible, and the doctor confirms that the radiographs are NOT SATISFACTORY, proceed to point 9.
9. Turn the patient into a prone position (lying on the abdomen) and take a prone abdomen view (ABDOMEN 7.3) 15 minutes after FILM 3; that is 25 minutes after the contrast injection was given—FILM 3A. FILM 3A, page 28
10. Turn the patient back into supine position (lying on his back).

ABDOMEN 7.4

11. Take a urinary bladder and inner pelvis view (ABDOMEN 6) with the bladder full—FILM 4. FILM 4, page 29
12. Ask the patient to empty the bladder (urinate), or realease the catheter, and take a second view—FILM 4A. FILM 4A, page 29
13. Show all the radiographs to the doctor; keep the patient on the X-ray table until they have been checked.

REMEMBER, when developing the films, to mark the time on each one so that the interval between the injection and the exposure is clear.
Use **R**ight and **L**eft markers.

INTRAVENOUS UROGRAPHY:
EXAMINATIONS OF THE KIDNEYS, URETERS, AND BLADDER

1. Ask the patient to empty the bladder before lying on the table. If there is a catheter in the bladder, open the catheter and drain the urine into a container.
2. Take FILM 1, abdomen and pelvis with the patient lying supine (ABDOMEN 5).
   Use a **R**ight or **L**eft marker
3. If the pelvis is not completely visible on the radiograph adjust the X-ray stand and take FILM 1A, urinary bladder and inner pelvis view (ABDOMEN 6).

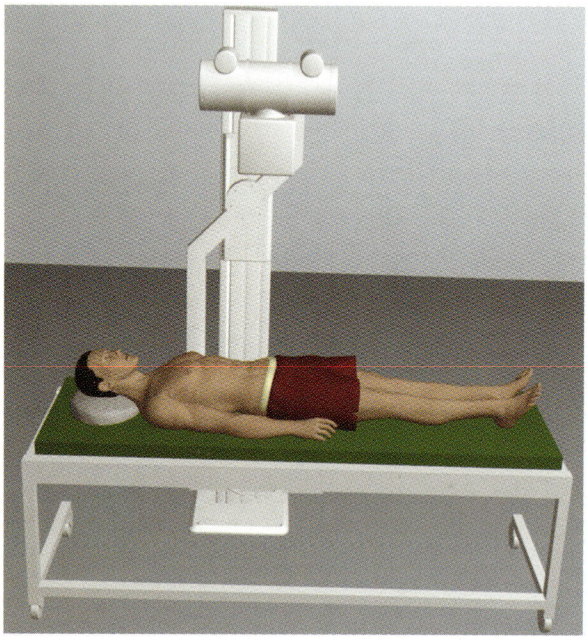

Position ABDOMEN 5

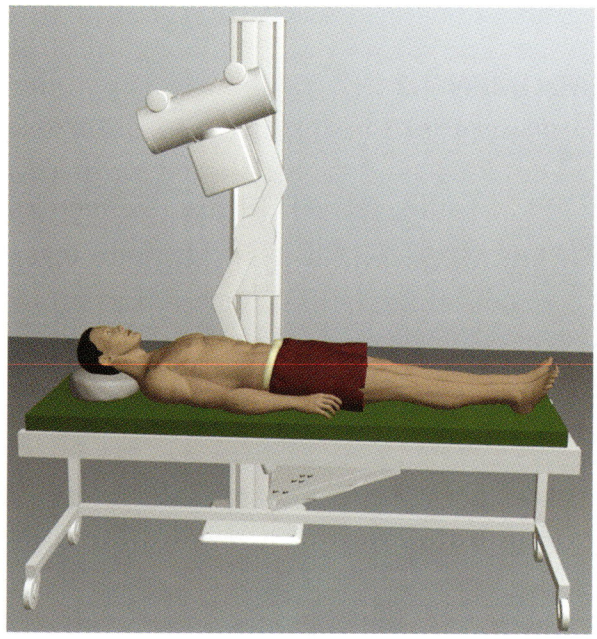

Position ABDOMEN 6

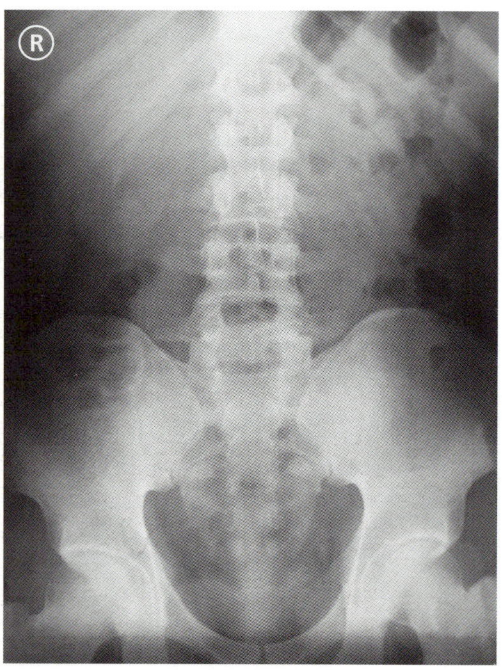

FILM 1

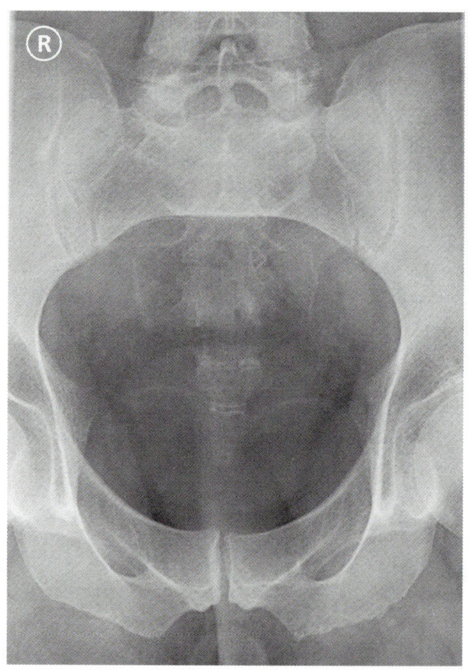

FILM 1A

Intravenous urography (continued)

4. When FILM 1 (and FILM 1A if it has been necessary to take it) have been checked by the doctor, the doctor gives the patient the contrast injection.
5. MAKE A NOTE OF THE TIME THE INJECTION IS GIVEN in the patients record.
6. As soon as the injection is given make sure the doctor moves behind the control screen or out of the X-ray room. Take FILM 2, a urinary tract survey with the patient lying supine (ABDOMEN 5).
7. AFTER 10 MINUTES take FILM 3, another urinary tract survey with the patient lying supine (ABDOMEN 5).

8a. SHOW FILM 2 AND FILM 3 TO THE DOCTOR. The kidneys, ureters and bladder should be visible. When the doctor has seen the films, turn to the next page.

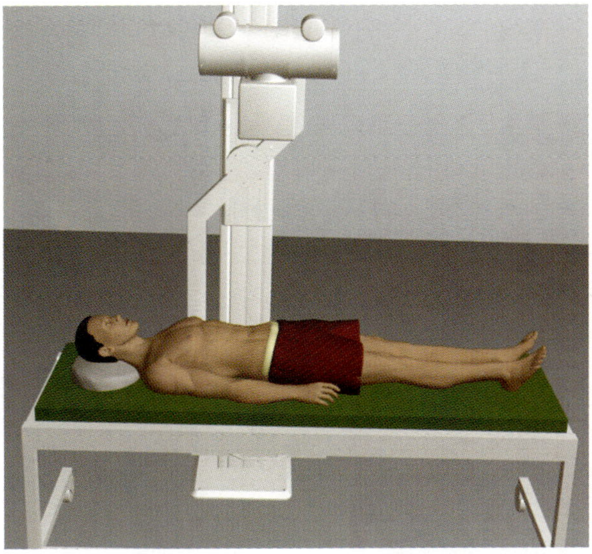

Position ABDOMEN 5

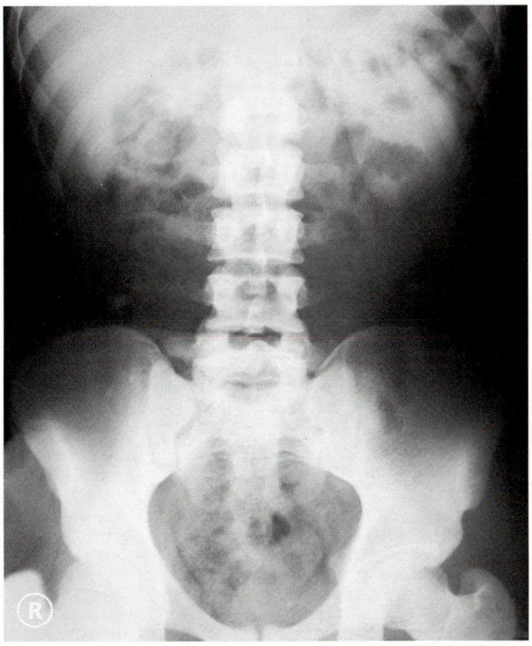

FILM 2

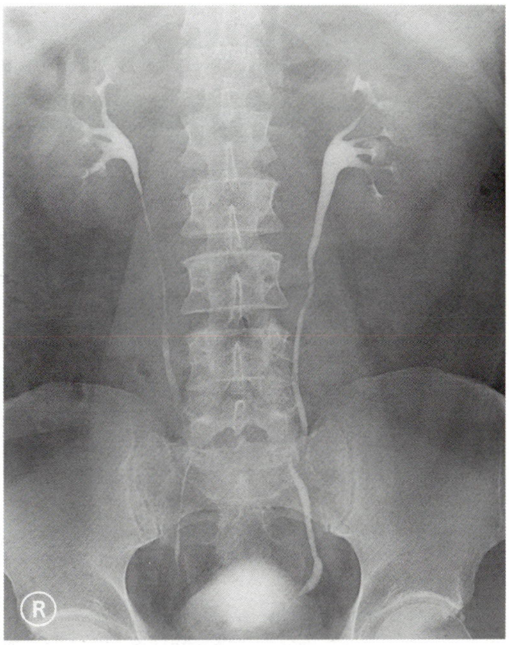

FILM 3

Intravenous urography (continued)

8b. If the doctor confirms that the films (FILM 2 and FILM 3) are SATISFACTORY, turn to the next page and take FILM 4.

8c. If the doctor says that the films are NOT SATISFACTORY:

9a. Turn the patient into a prone position (lying on the abdomen as shown below) and make sure the tube is pointing on the centre of the lumbar spine. Use the same the position of the machine (stand) and exposure. Make sure that the **L** or **R** marker is correctly positioned when the patient is turned around to the prone position.

9b. 25 minutes after the contrast injection was given take FILM 3A (PRONE ABDOMEN).

10. Check that the film is satisfactory. Turn the patient back into supine position (lying on his back). Go to the next page and take FILM 4.

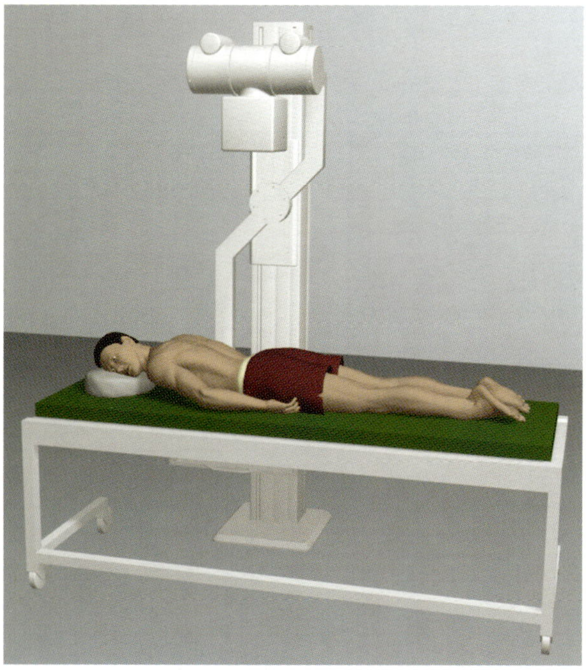

Position PRONE ABDOMEN

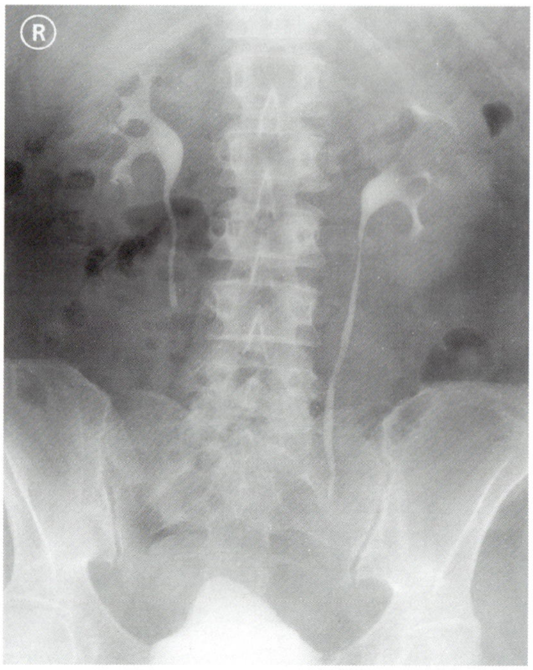

FILM 3A

Intravenous urography (continued) **bladder film**

11a. Take FILM 4 (ABDOMEN 6) with the bladder full.

11b. Check the quality of the film.

12a. A soon as a SATISFACTORY film is obtained, send the patient to empty the bladder (urinate), or release the catheter.

12b. Take FILM 4A (ABDOMEN 6).

13. Show all the films to the doctor; keep the patient on the X-ray table until they have been checked.

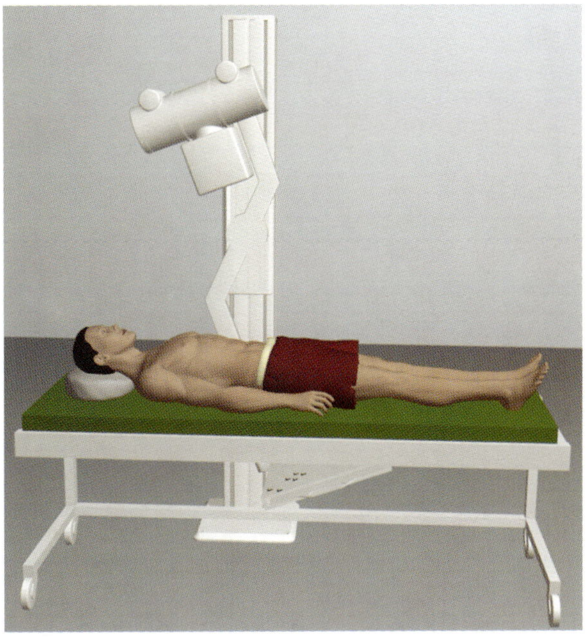

Position ABDOMEN 6

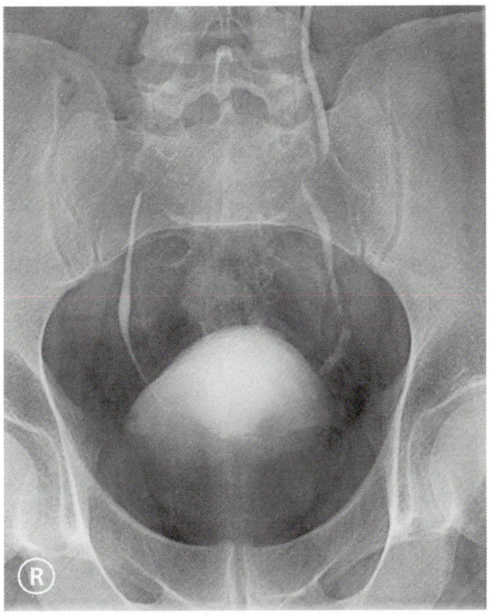

FILM 4

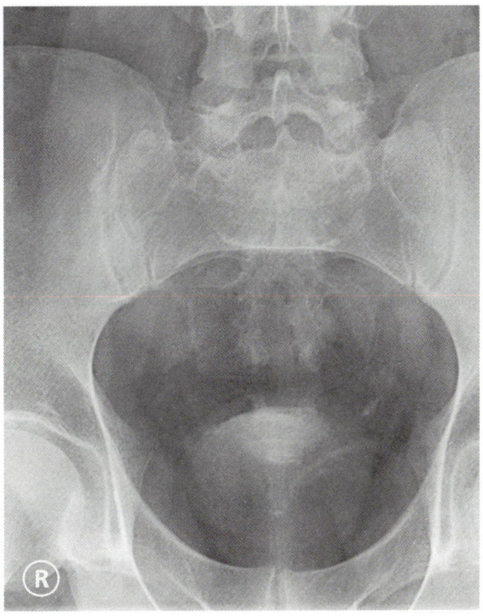

FILM 4A

PREGNANCY LATERAL Standing erect BASIC

Take this view when obstructed labour (disproportion) is suspected, but NOT before the 37th week of pregnancy.
Do not use this examination if ultrasound is available.

Cassette speed
Cassette with screen-film combination, nominal speed 200/400 in the cassette holder

Cassette size
35×43 cm (14×17 inches)

Exposure values	mAs	
90 kV	"blue" system 200	"green" system 400/500
Average	160	63
Range	100–200	40–80

1. The patient must EMPTY HER BLADDER BEFORE THE X-RAY is taken.
2. Bring in the patient, put the cassette in the cassette holder. Collimate to the format.
3. Tell the patient to stand with the left side against the cassette holder. Place a measuring-rod between the legs, as shown. Centre. Collimate further, if possible.
4. Tell the patient to STOP breathing. Expose.
5. Tell the patient to breathe normally.

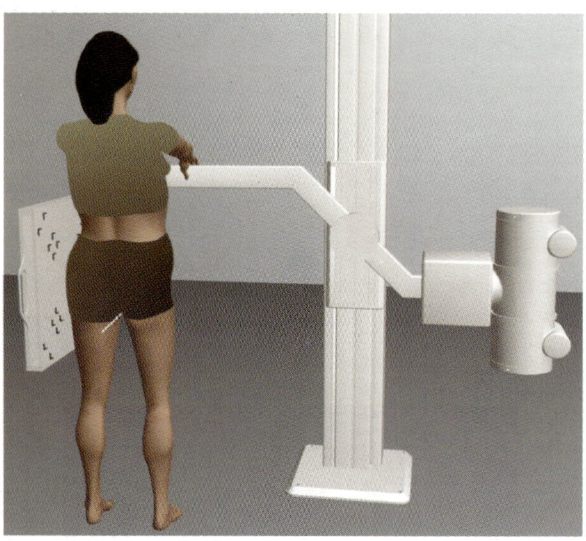

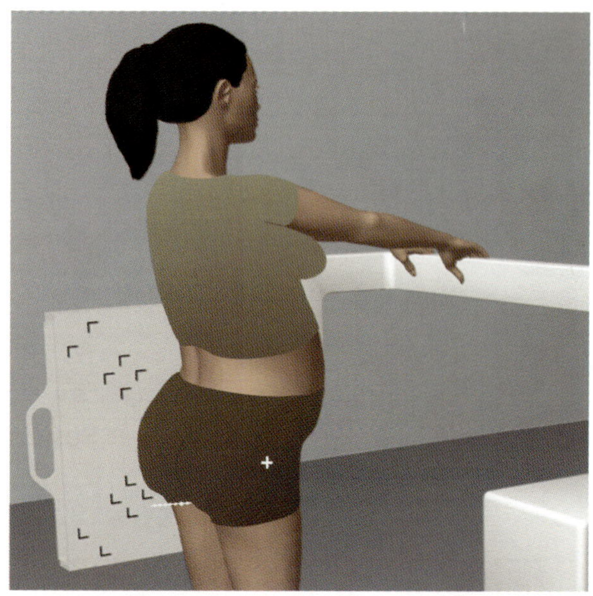

Comment

Make sure the symphysis is shown on the film.

Measuring-rod

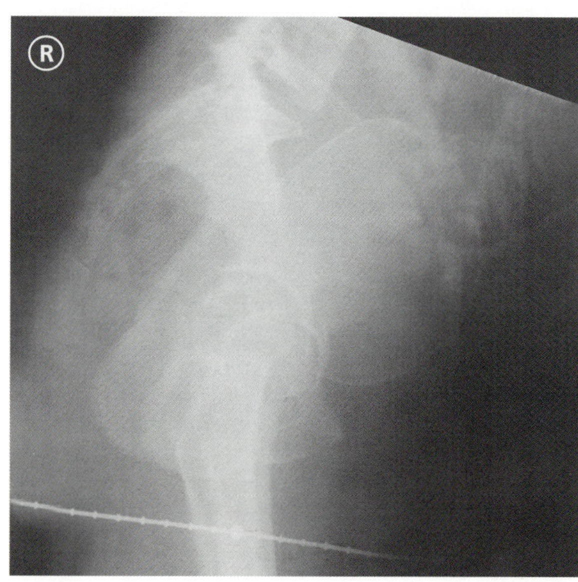

PREGNANCY PA (or AP) Prone with support under the pelvis BASIC

Take this view when obstructed labour (disproportion) is suspected, but NOT before the 37th week of pregnancy

Do not use this examination if ultrasound is available.

Cassette speed
Cassette with screen-film combination, nominal speed 200/400 in the cassette holder

Cassette size
35×43 cm (14×17 inches)
Use a **R**ight or **L**eft marker

Exposure values	mAs	
90 kV	"blue" system 200	"green" system 400/500
Average	160	63
Range	100–200	40–80

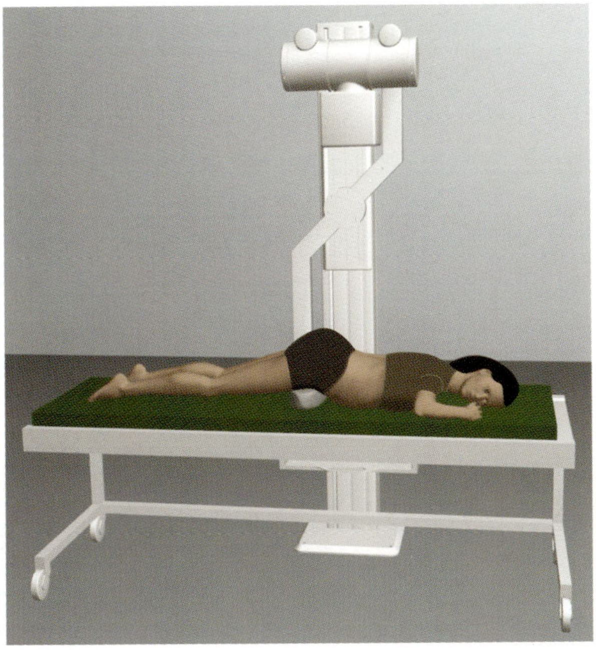

1. The patient must EMPTY HER BLADDER BEFORE THE X-RAY is taken.
2. Bring in the patient, put the cassette in the cassette holder. Collimate to the format.
3. Position the patient as shown (if the patient finds it impossible to lie prone use the supine position). Centre. Collimate further, if possible. Make sure that the **R** or **L** marker is correctly positioned when the patient is in the prone position.
4. Tell the patient to STOP breathing. Expose.
5. Tell the patient to breathe normally.

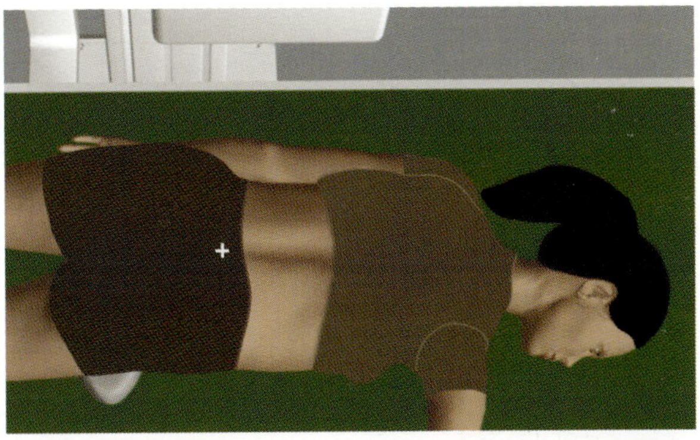

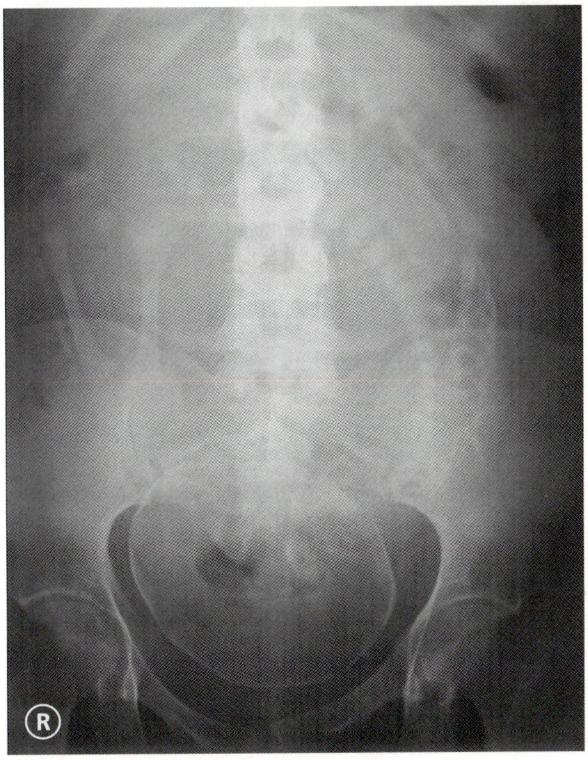

Head

SKULL

X-rays of the skull are always taken with the patient lying down.

1. Skull PA, page 34.
   (Do not use for infants or children – use HEAD 2)
   NEVER USE this position when there is a possibility that the facial bones may be fractured or when the patient is unconcious.
2. Skull AP, page 35.
3. Skull (occiput) semiaxial (Towne's projection), page 36.
4. Skull lateral, page 37.

SINUSES, FACE, AND NOSE

These examinations are unreliable under the age of 7 years

Patient sitting

5. Sinuses and face semiaxial, or nose PA, page 38.
6. Sinuses and face PA, page 39.
7. Sinuses, face, or nose lateral, page 40.

Patient lying down, unable to sit

Sinuses face, or nose AP – use Skull AP (HEAD 2, page 35)

Sinuses, face, or nose lateral – use Skull lateral (HEAD 4, page 37)

MANDIBLE

Patient sitting

8. Mandible PA, page 41.
9. Mandible oblique lateral, page 42.

Patient lying down, unable to sit

10. Mandible AP, page 43.
11. Mandible oblique lateral, page 44.

SKULL PA **Prone – vertical beam angled 20° as shown** BASIC

Never use when there is a possibility that the facial bones may be fractured or when the patient is unconscious. Use HEAD 3 instead.

Cassette speed
Cassette with screen-film combination, nominal speed 200/400 in the cassette holder

Cassette size
24×30 cm (10×12 inches)
Use a **R**ight or **L**eft marker

Exposure values	mAs	
70 **kV**	"blue" system 200	"green" system 400
Average	100	50
Range	63–125	32–63

1. Bring in the patient, put the cassette in the cassette holder. Collimate to the format.
2. Remove dentures, earclips, hairgrips, or anything from the hair. Mattress for the body. Place hands under the chest. Place the forehead and the nose on the stretcher-table.
3. Center and collimate further, if possible.
4. Expose.

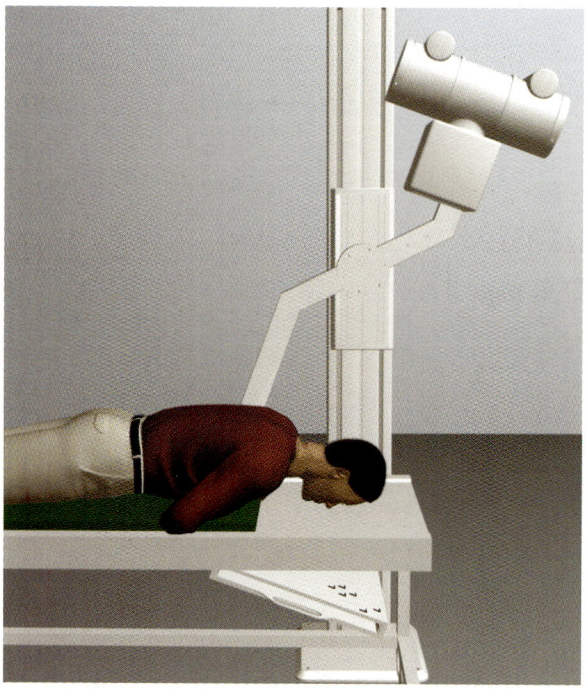

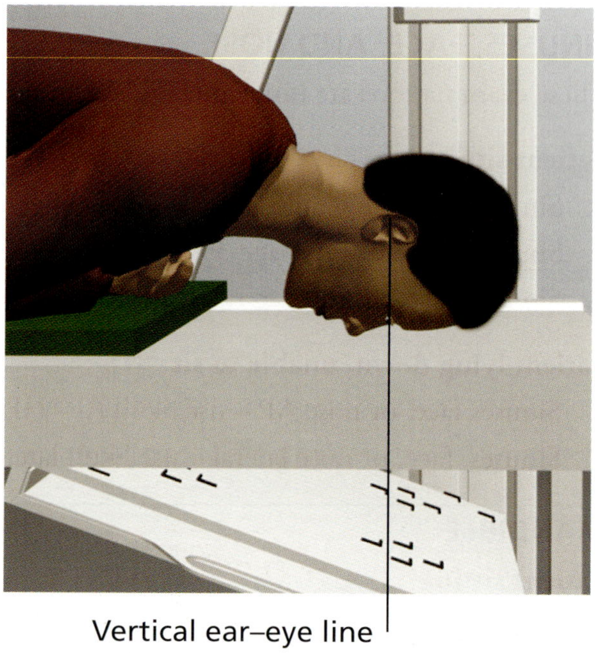

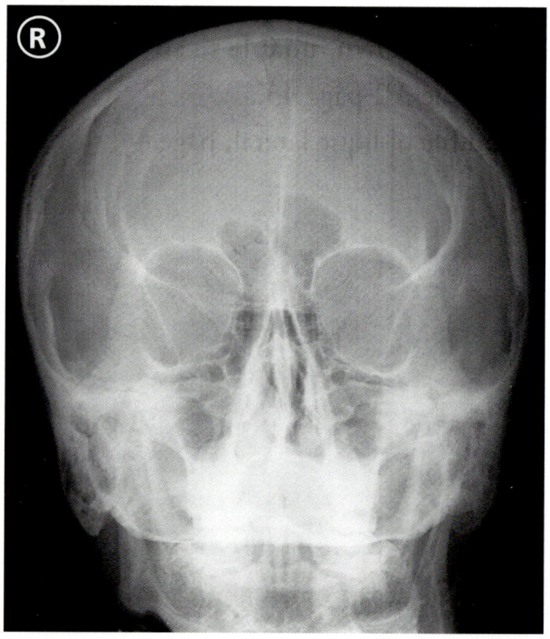

SKULL AP **Supine – vertical beam angled 20° as shown** ADDITIONAL

Use when the patient cannot be X-rayed in a prone position.

Cassette speed

Cassette with screen-film combination, nominal speed 200/400 in the cassette holder

Cassette size

24×30 cm (10×12 inches)

Use a **R**ight or **L**eft marker

Exposure values	**mAs**	
70 **kV**	"blue" system 200	"green" system 400
Average	100	50
Range	63–125	32–63

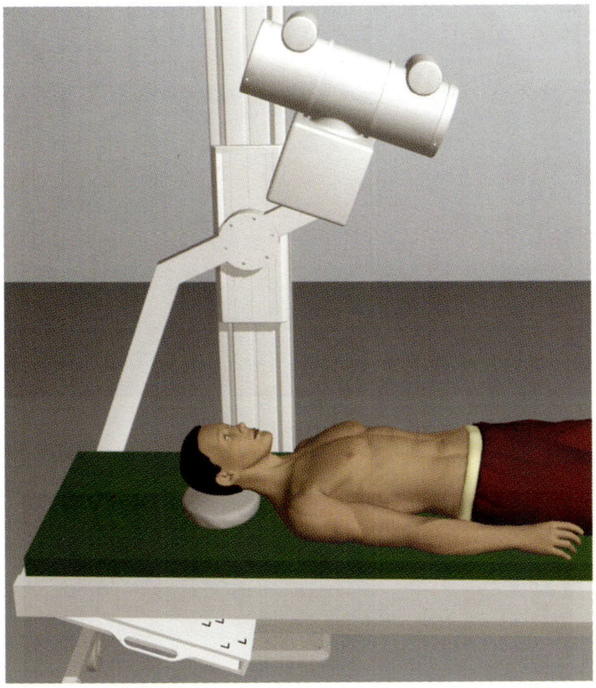

1. Bring in the patient, put the cassette in the cassette holder. Collimate to the format.
2. Remove dentures, earclips, hairgrips, or anything from the hair.
3. Mattress. The patient's head should lie flat raised on a thin radiolucent (e.g.foam rubber) pad. Do not use a pillow.
4. Center to the root of the nose between the eyes. Collimate further, if possible.
5. Expose.

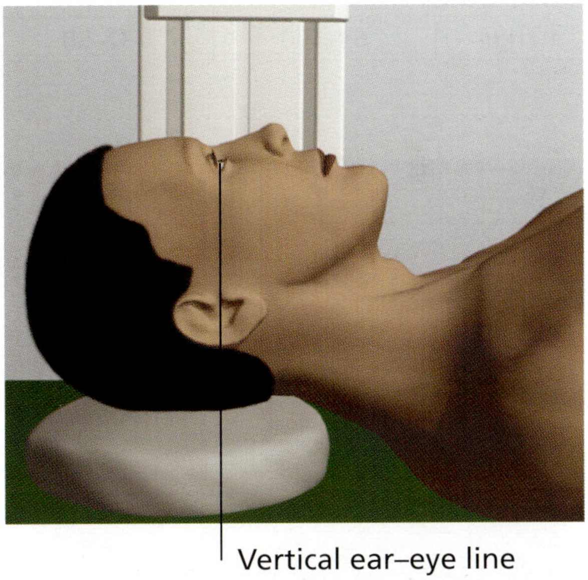

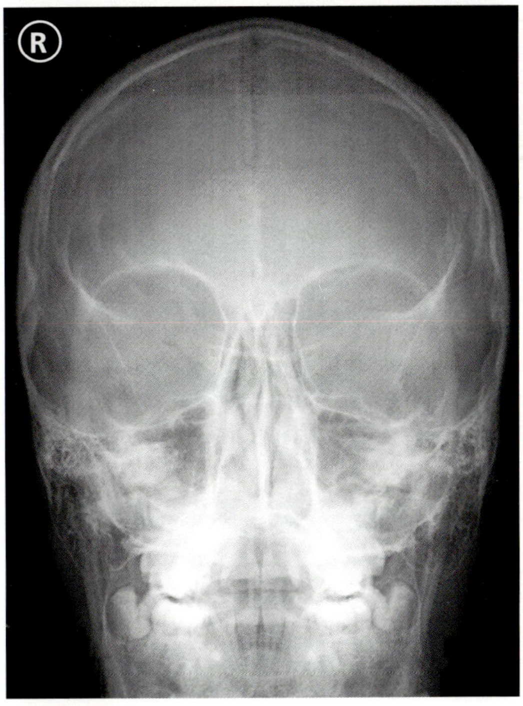

SKULL (OCCIPUT) SEMIAXIAL (TOWNE'S PROJECTION) Supine – vertical beam angled 30° as shown ADDITIONAL

Cassette speed
Cassette with screen-film combination, nominal speed 200/400 in the cassette holder

Cassette size
24×30 cm (10×12 inches)
Use a **R**ight or **L**eft marker

Exposure values	mAs	
70 **kV**	"blue" system 200	"green" system 400
Average	80	40
Range	63–100	32–50

1. Bring in the patient, put the cassette in the cassette holder. Collimate to the format.
2. Remove dentures, earclips, hairgrips, or anything from the hair.
3. Mattress. The patient's head should lie flat raised on a thin radiolucent (e.g. foam rubber) pad. Do not use a regular pillow.
4. Center to the top of the head 7–8 cm from the root of the nose.
5. Collimate further, if possible.
6. Expose.

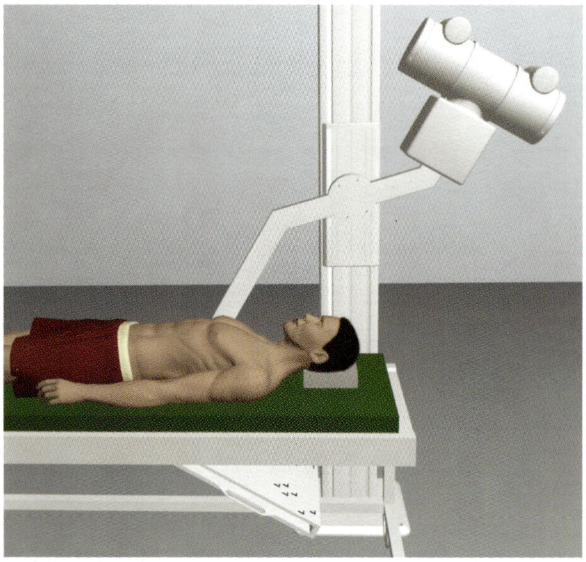

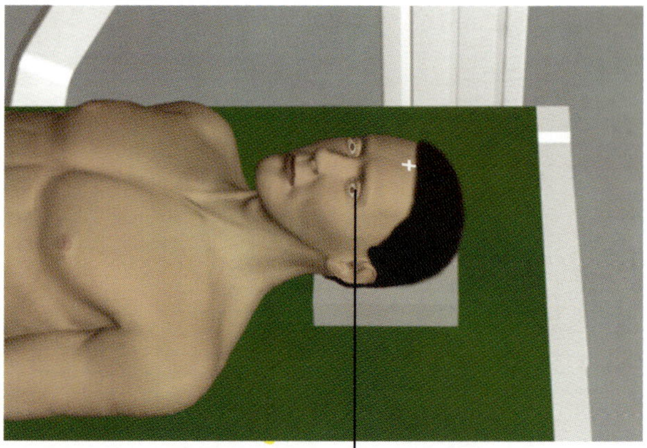

Vertical ear–eye line

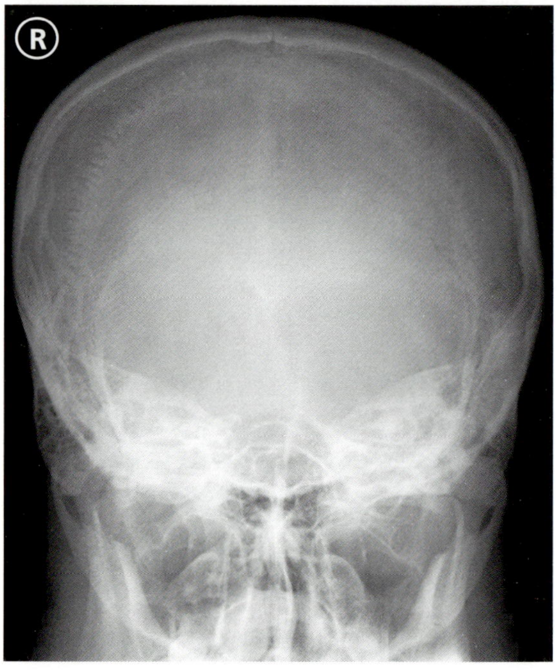

SKULL LATERAL Supine – horizontal beam BASIC

Cassette speed
Cassette with screen-film combination, nominal speed 200/400 in the cassette holder

Cassette size
24×30 cm (10×12 inches)
Use a **R**ight or **L**eft marker to denote which side of the head that is close to the cassette

Exposure values	mAs	
70 **kV**	"blue" system 200	"green" system 400
Average	32	16
Range	25–40	12.5–20

1. Bring in the patient, put the cassette in the cassette holder. Collimate to the format.
2. Remove dentures, earclips, hairgrips, or anything from the hair.
3. Mattress. The patient's head should lie flat raised on a thin radiolucent (e.g. foam rubber) pad. Do not use a regular pillow.
4. The line from the outer corner of the eye to the ear opening shall be at right angle to the examination table.
5. Center as shown.
   Collimate further, if possible.
6. Expose.

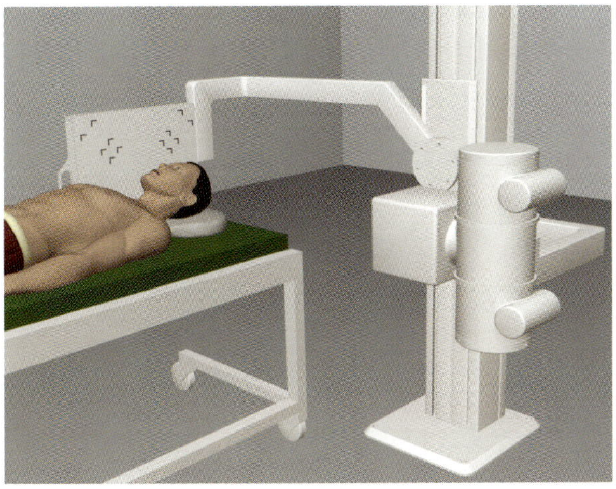

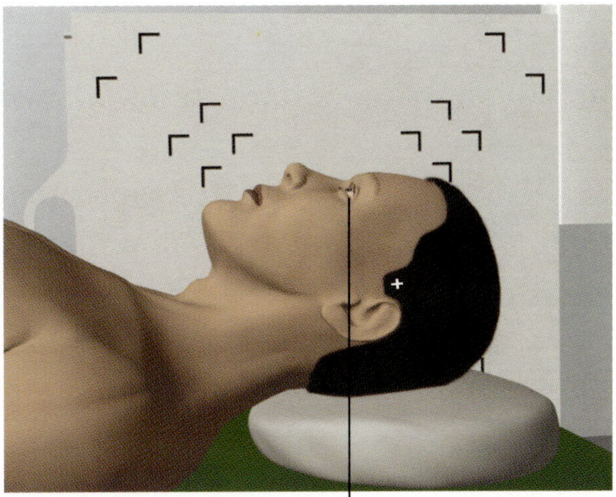

Vertical ear–eye line

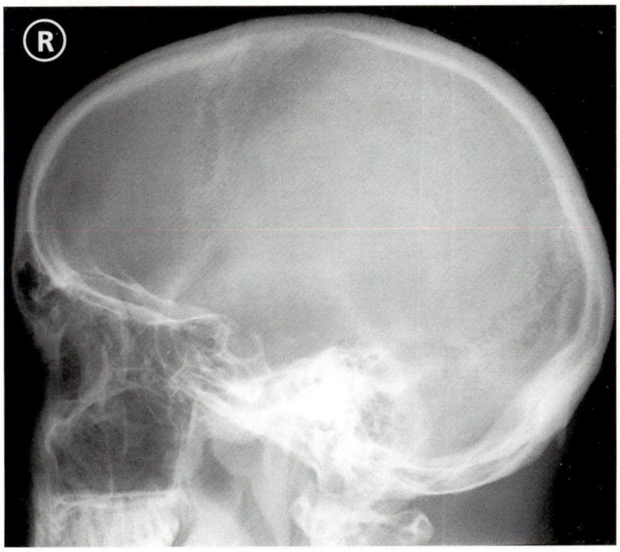

Front and back of skull must be visible

SINUSES and FACE SEMIAXIAL or NOSE PA Sitting erect BASIC

If the patient is unable to sit, use the supine position (HEAD 3).
Use this view when only one view of the sinuses is requested.
Under the age of 7 years x-ray of the sinuses is unreliable for infection.

Cassette speed
Cassette with screen-film combination, nominal speed 200/400 in the cassette holder

Cassette size
18×24 cm (8×10 inches) for sinus
24×30 cm (10×12 inches) for face
Use a **R**ight or **L**eft marker

Exposure values	mAs	
80 **kV**	"blue" system 200	"green" system 400/450
Average	63	25
Range	50–80	20–32

1. Bring in the patient, put the cassette in the cassette holder. Collimate to the format.
2. Remove dentures, hairgrips, or anything from the hair.
3. Position the patient. Tell the patient to open the mouth as widely as possible and place the chin against the cassette holder. Tilt the patient's head back 45°.
4. Center as shown.
   Collimate further, if possible.
5. Expose.

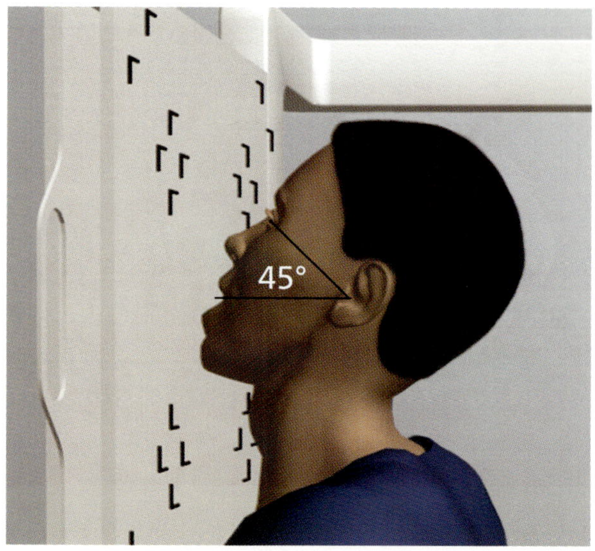

45°-line – ear opening to lateral corner of the eye

Horizontal line – ear opening to mouth

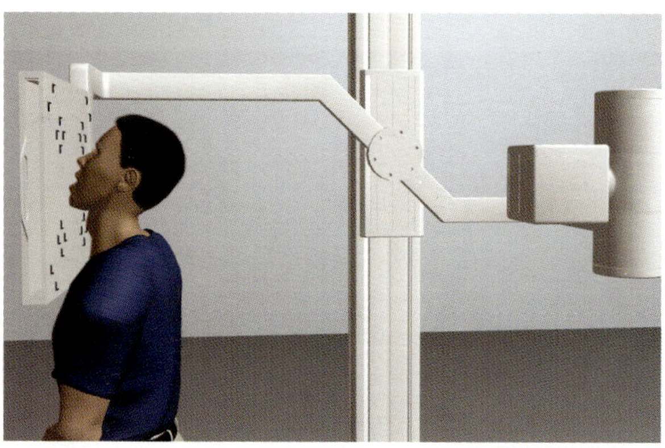

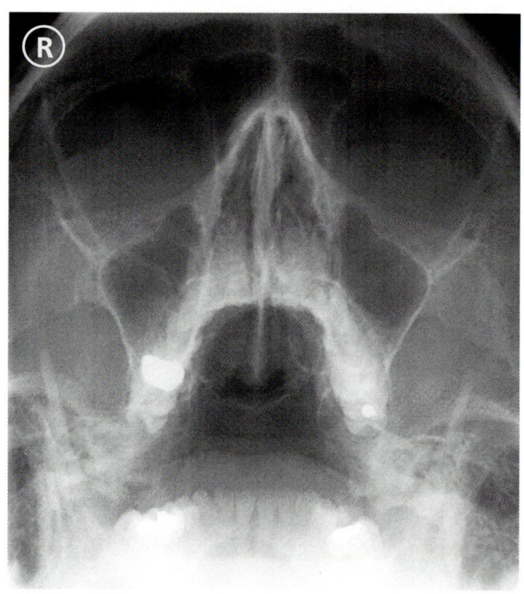

SINUSES and FACE PA Sitting erect BASIC (face) ADDITIONAL (sinuses)

If ONLY ONE VIEW of the sinuses is requested by the doctor, use HEAD 5

Cassette speed
Cassette with screen-film combination, nominal speed 200/400 in the cassette holder

Cassette size
18×24 cm (8×10 inches) for sinus
24×30 cm (10×12 inches) for face
Use a **R**ight or **L**eft marker

Exposure values	mAs	
80 kV	"blue" system 200	"green" system 400/450
Average	50	20
Range	40–63	16–25

1. Bring in the patient, put the cassette in the cassette holder. Collimate to the format.
2. Remove dentures, hairgrips, or anything from the hair.
3. Position the patient. The line between the lower bony edge of the eye and the ear opening must be at a right angle to the cassette holder.
4. Center corresponding to the root of the nose between the eyes.
   Collimate further, if possible.
5. Expose.

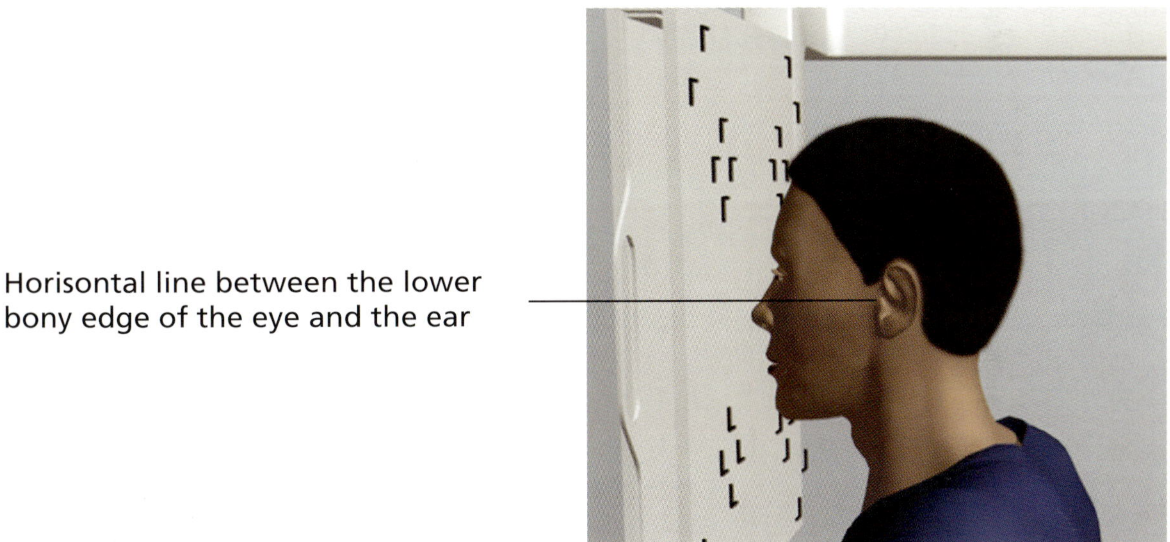

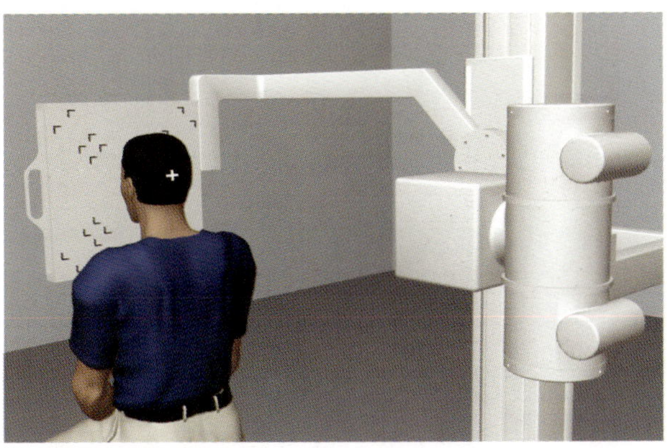

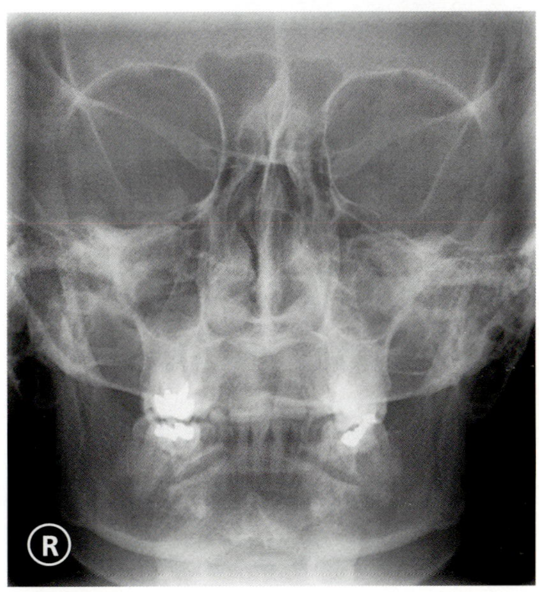

SINUSES, FACE or **NOSE LATERAL** **Sitting erect**

BASIC (nose) ADDITIONAL (sinuses and face)

If the patient is unable to sit, use the supine position (HEAD 4).
Do not use for children under 7 years of age, except for trauma or suspected tumors.

Cassette speed
Cassette with screen-film combination, nominal speed 100/200/400 in the cassette holder

Cassette size
18×24 cm (8×10 inches) for sinus
24×30 cm (10×12 inches) for face

Exposure values	mAs	
80 **kV**	"blue" system 200	"green" system 400/450
Average	12.5	5
Nose 53 **kV**	"blue" system 200	"green" system 100/63
Average	4	8

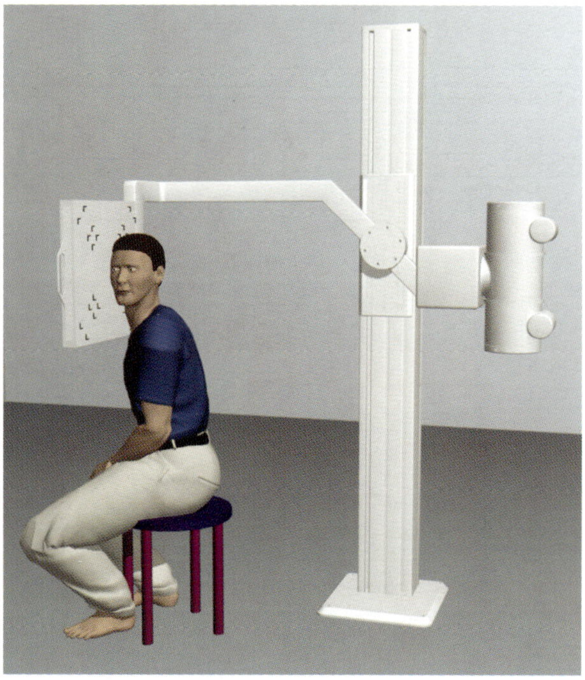

1. Bring in the patient, put the cassette in the cassette holder. Collimate to the format.
2. Remove dentures, earclips, hairgrips, or anything from the hair.
3. Position the right side of the patient's head next to the cassette holder.
4. Center as shown.
   Collimate further, if possible.
5. Expose.

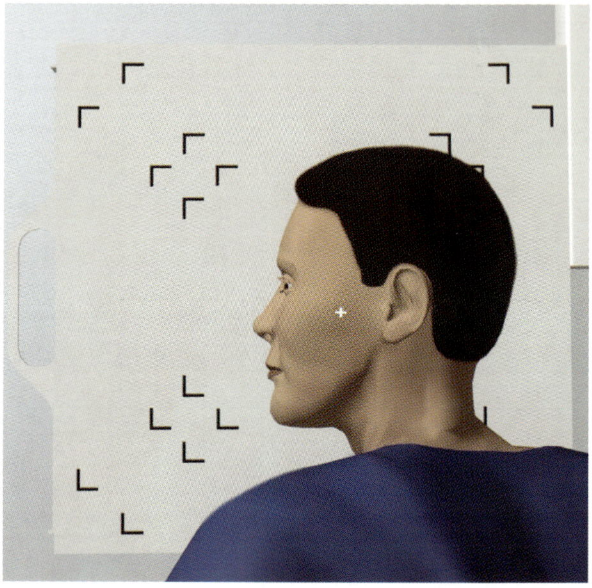

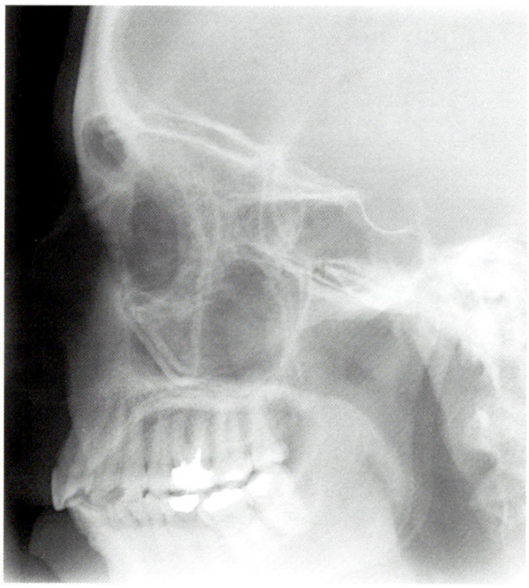

MANDIBLE PA Sitting erect BASIC

Cassette speed
Cassette with screen-film combination, nominal speed 200/400 in the cassette holder

Cassette size
24×30 cm (10×12 inches)
Use a **R**ight or **L**eft marker

Exposure values	"blue" system 200	"green" system 400
70 **kV**	63 **mAs**	32 **mAs**

1. Bring in the patient, put the cassette in the cassette holder. Collimate to the format.
2. Remove dentures, hairgrips, or anything from the hair.
3. Tell the patient to open the mouth as widely as possible and place the forehead and nose against the cassette holder. The line from the outer corner of the eye to the ear opening shall be at right angle to the cassette holder.
4. Center as shown.
   Collimate further, if possible.
5. Expose.

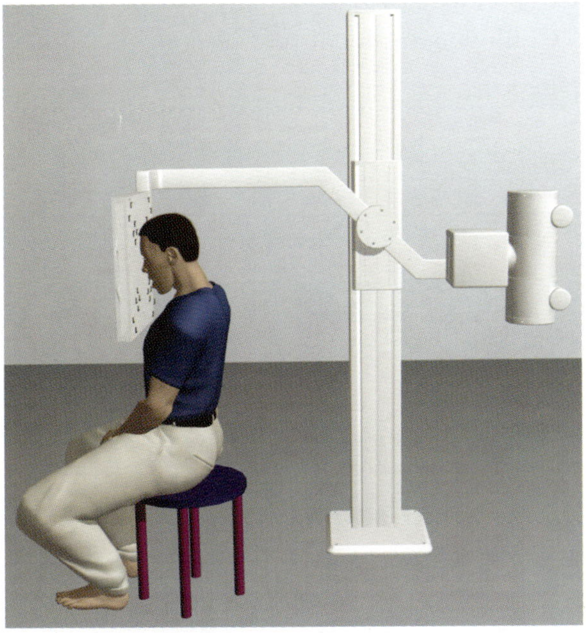

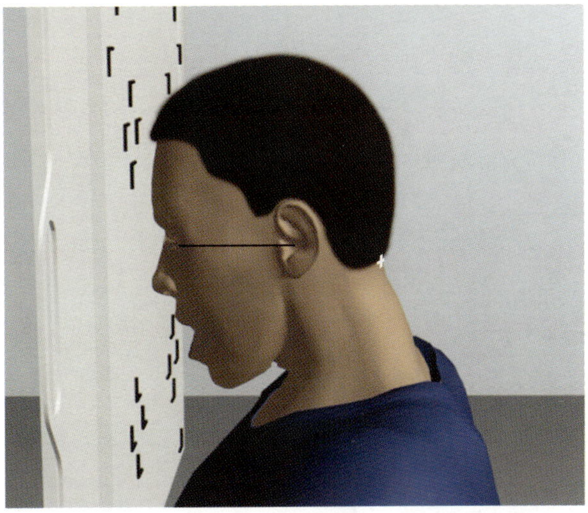

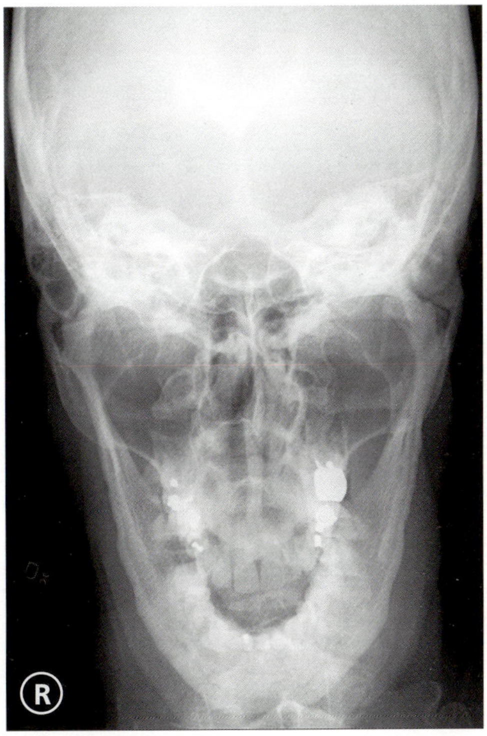

MANDIBLE OBLIQUE LATERAL Sitting erect (right or left) – horizontal beam angled 15° as shown BASIC

Cassette speed
Cassette with screen-film combination, nominal speed 200/400 in the cassette holder

Cassette size
18×24 cm (8×10 inches)
Use a **R**ight or **L**eft marker

Exposure values	"blue" system 200	"green" system 400
70 **kV**	12.5 **mAs**	6.3 **mAs**

1. Bring in the patient, put the cassette in the cassette holder. Collimate to the format.
2. Remove dentures, hairgrips, or anything from the hair.
3. Angle the X-ray tube 15° as shown.
4. Ask the patient to sit with the side of the head to be X-rayed nearest to the cassette holder. (Right side shown).
5. Tilt the head inwards 15° as shown, so that the head and shoulder rest against the cassette holder.
6. Center as shown.
   Collimate further, if possible.
7. Expose.

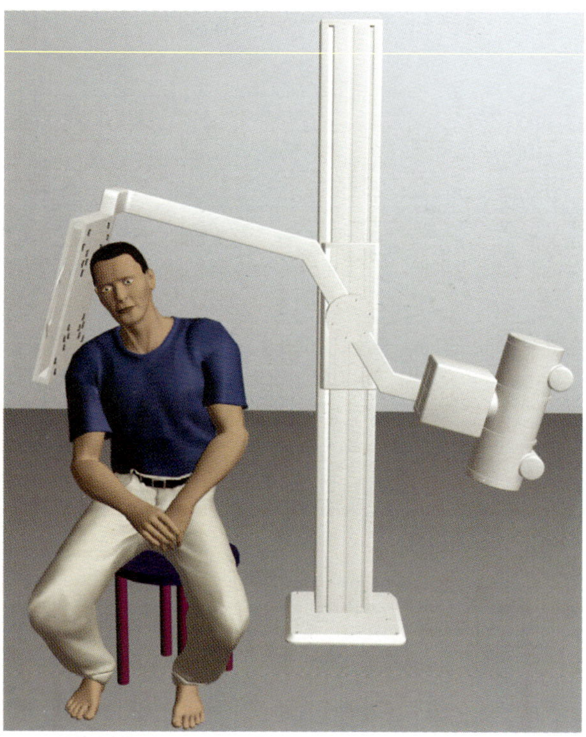

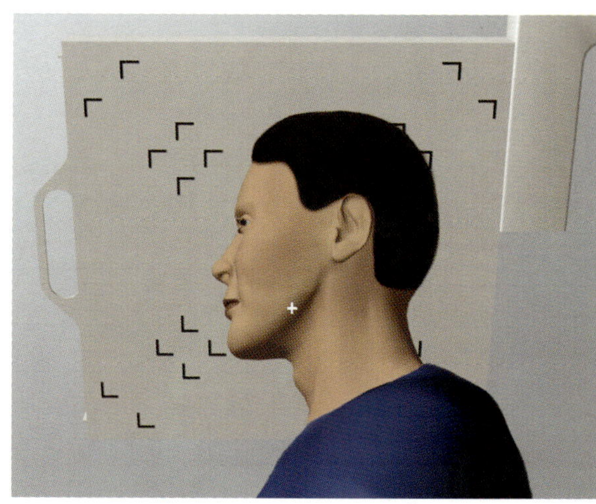

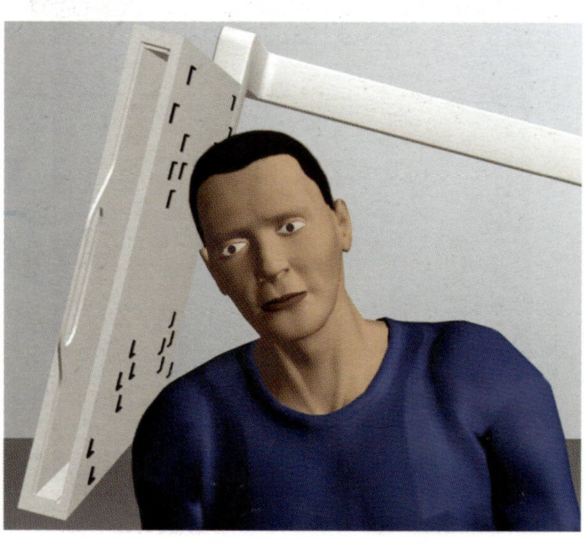

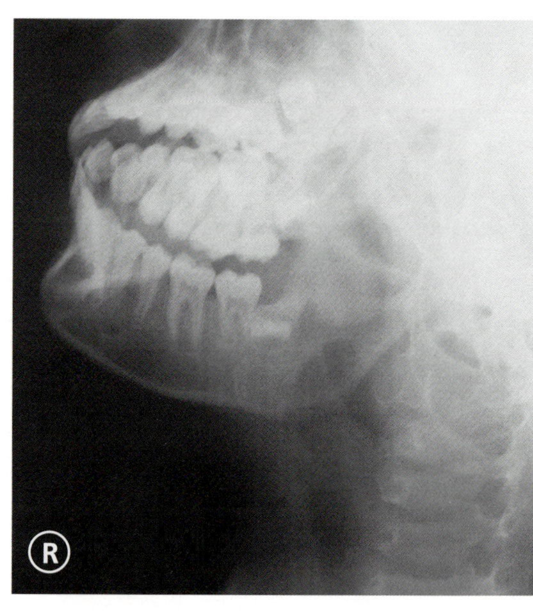

MANDIBLE AP Supine – vertical beam angled 30° as shown ADDITIONAL

Cassette speed
Cassette with screen-film combination, nominal speed 200/400 in the cassette holder

Cassette size
24×30 cm (10×12 inches)
Use a **R**ight or **L**eft marker

Exposure values	"blue" system 200	"green" system 400
70 **kV**	63 **mAs**	32 **mAs**

1. Bring in the patient, put the cassette in the cassette holder. Collimate to the format.
2. Remove dentures, hairgrips, or anything from the hair.
3. Tell the patient to open the mouth as widely as possible. If the patient is unable to keep the mouth open place a wedge of soft wood or cork between upper and lower row of teeth or gums. The line between the lower bony edge of the eye and the ear opening must be at a right angle to the the examination table.
4. Center as shown.
   Collimate further, if possible.
5. Expose. Remove wedge of cork.

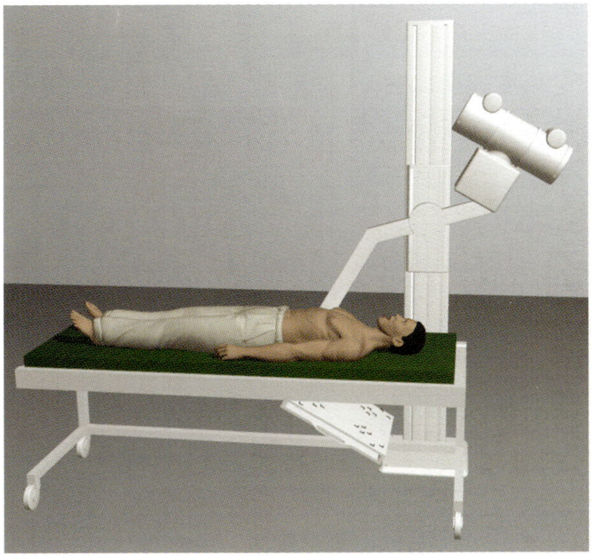

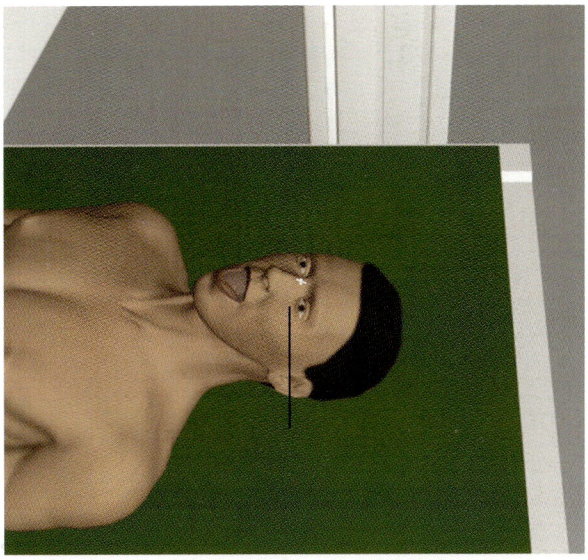

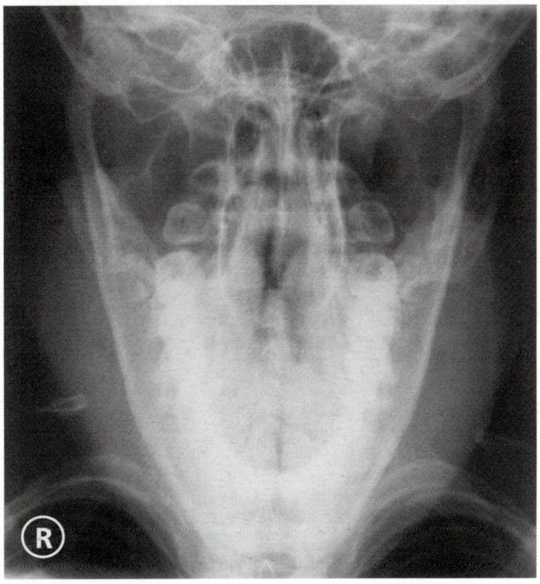

MANDIBLE OBLIQUE LATERAL Lying on the side (right or left) – vertical beam angled 15° as shown ADDITIONAL

Cassette speed
Cassette with screen-film combination, nominal speed 200/400 in the cassette holder

Cassette size
18×24 cm (8×10 inches)
Use a **R**ight or **L**eft marker

Exposure values	"blue" system 200	"green" system 400
70 **kV**	12.5 **mAs**	6.3 **mAs**

1. Bring in the patient, put the cassette in the cassette holder. Collimate to the format.
2. Remove dentures, hairgrips, earrings, or anything from the hair.
3. Angle the X-ray tube 15° as shown.
4. Position the patient with the side to be X-rayed nearest to the table. (Right side shown).
5. Tilt the patient's head 15° as shown.
6. Center as shown.
   Collimate further, if possible.
7. Expose.

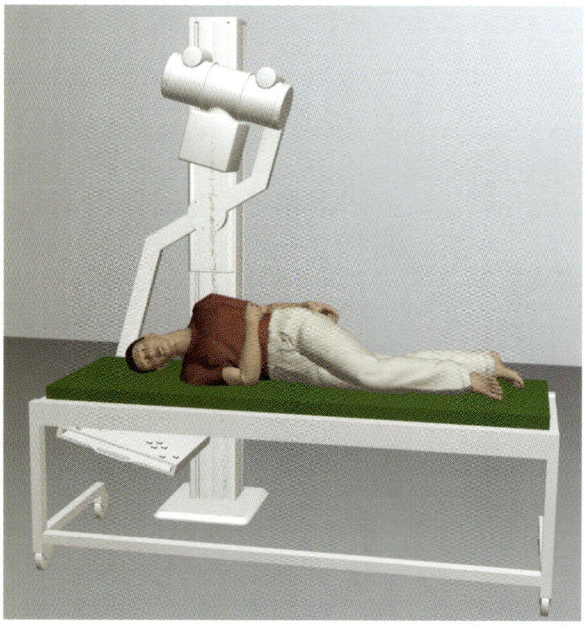

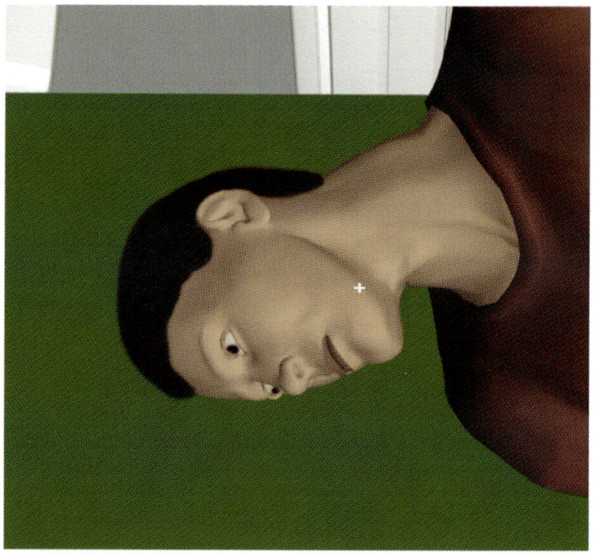

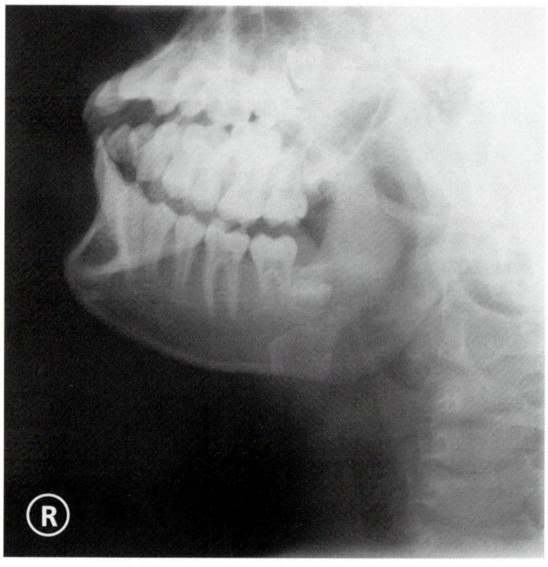

Spine

CERVICAL SPINE

Patients able to sit

1. Cervical spine PA, page 46.
2. Cervical spine lateral, page 47.
3. Cervical spine oblique, page 48.

Patients lying down, unable to sit

4. Cervical spine AP – after injury, page 49.
5. Cervical spine lateral – after injury, page 50.
6. Odontoid process AP – first and second cervical vertebrae, page 51.

CERVICOTHORACIC REGION

7. Cervico-thoracic region lateral, page 52.
   When the patient has been injured, keep the patient lying on her/his back

THORACIC SPINE

8. Thoracic spine AP, page 53.
9. Thoracic spine lateral, page 54.

LUMBOSACRAL SPINE

10. Lumbar spine AP, page 55.
11. Lumbar spine lateral, page 56.
12. Lumbar spine lateral – after injury, page 57.
    Use ONLY after injury
13. Sacrum AP – lumbosacral junction and sacroiliac joints, page 58.
14. Lumbosacral junction lateral, page 59.

CERVICAL SPINE PA (or AP) Sitting erect BASIC

After injury, see SPINE 4

Cassette speed
Cassette with screen-film combination, nominal speed 200/400 in the cassette holder

Cassette size
18×24 cm (8×10 inches)
Use a **R**ight or **L**eft marker

Exposure values	mAs	
70 kV	"blue" system 200	"green" system 400
Average	25	12.5
Range	20–50	10–25

1. Bring in the patient, put the cassette in the cassette holder. Collimate to the format.
2. Remove necklace, hairgrips and anything else from the hair.
3. Tell the patient to place the chin against the cassette holder. The knob at the back of the head should be level with the chin (lower jaw).
4. Center and collimate further, if possible. Tell the patient to stop breathing.
5. Expose. Tell the patient to breathe normally.

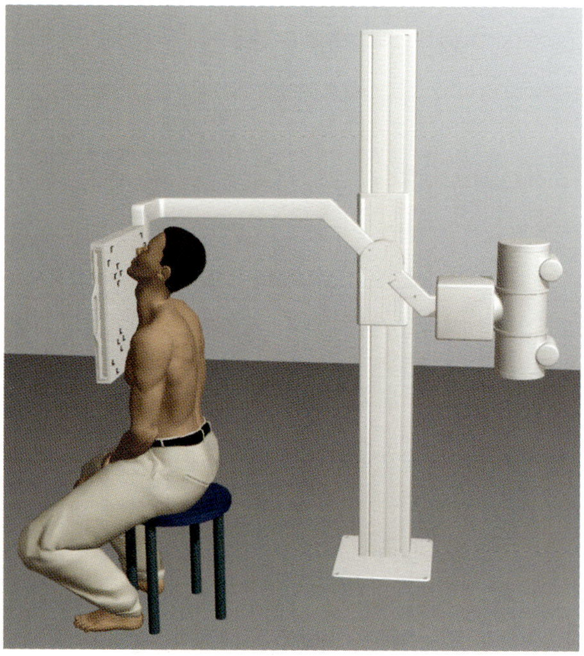

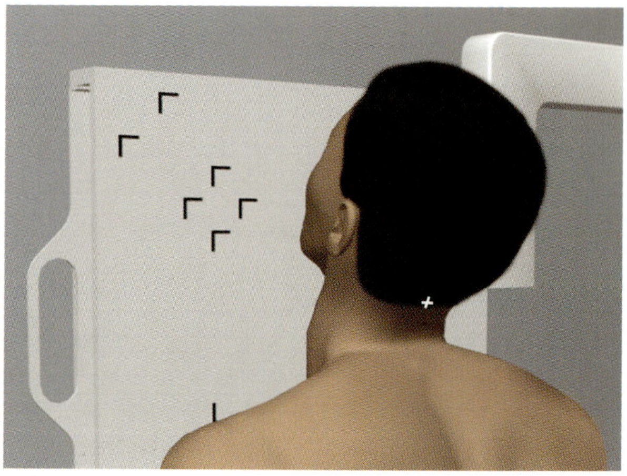

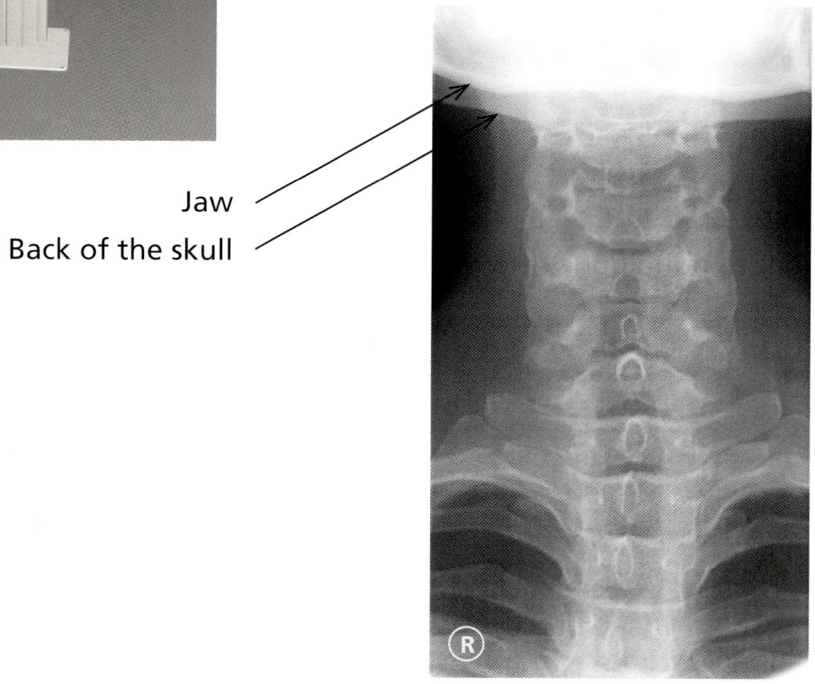

CERVICAL SPINE LATERAL Sitting erect BASIC

Cassette speed
Cassette with screen-film combination, nominal speed 200/400 in the cassette holder

Cassette size
18×24 cm (8×10 inches)

Exposure values	mAs	
70 kV	"blue" system 200	"green" system 400
Average	25	12.5
Range	20–50	10–25

1. Bring in the patient, put the cassette in the cassette holder. Collimate to the format.
2. Remove necklace, hairgrips and earclips and anything else from the hair.
3. Position the patient with the shoulder against the cassette holder. The shoulders as low as possible with the arms against the sides. If the patient is not injured put a 1 kg (2 lb) weight (not more) in each hand.
4. Center and collimate further, if possible. Tell the patient to stop breathing.
5. Expose. Tell the patient to breathe normally.

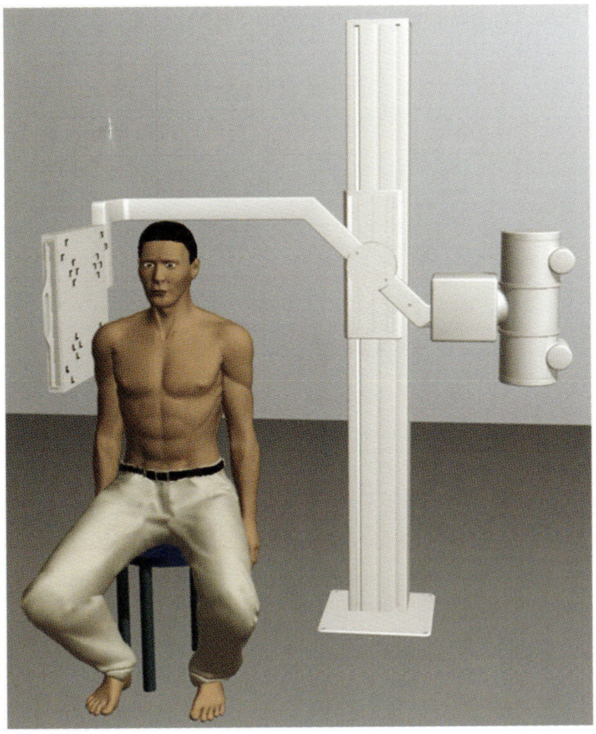

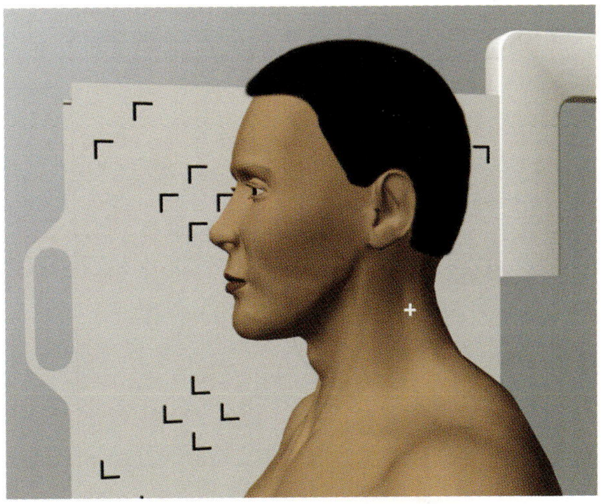

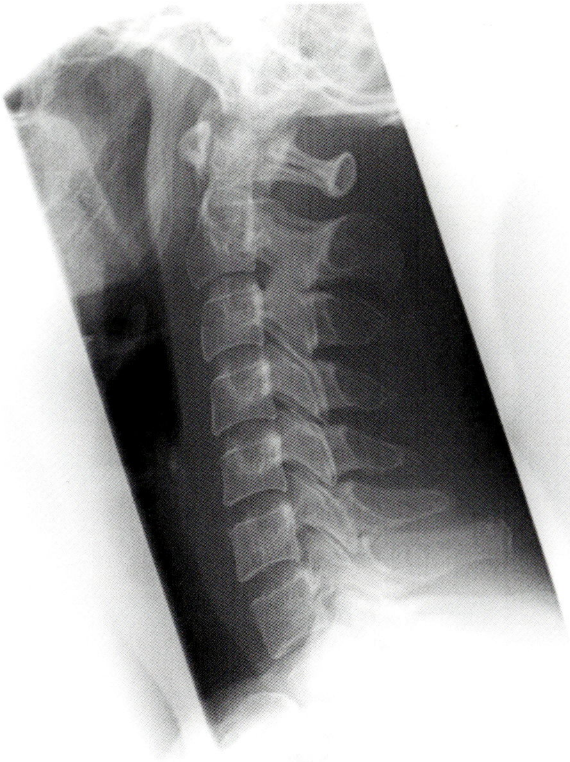

CERVICAL SPINE OBLIQUE Sitting erect ADDITIONAL

Do not use for children

Cassette speed
Cassette with screen-film combination, nominal speed 200/400 in the cassette holder

Cassette size
18×24 cm (8×10 inches)
Use a **R**ight **and L**eft marker

Exposure values	mAs	
70 kV	"blue" system 200	"green" system 400
Average	25	12.5
Range	20–50	10–25

1. Bring in the patient, put the cassette in the cassette holder. Collimate to the format.
2. Remove necklace, hairgrips, earclips and anything else from the hair.
3. Position the patient. Rotate the patient so that he is sitting at a 45° angle to the cassette holder.
4. Center and collimate further, if possible. Tell the patient to stop breathing.
5. Expose. Tell the patient to breathe normally.
6. Turn the patient and repeat for the other oblique view.

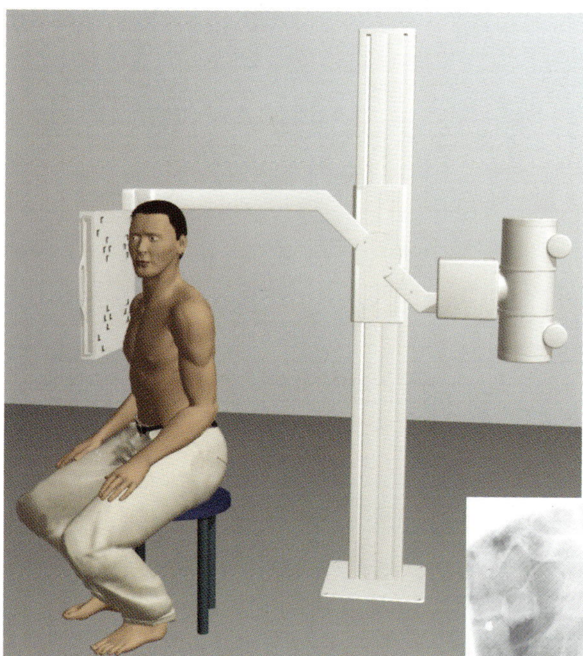

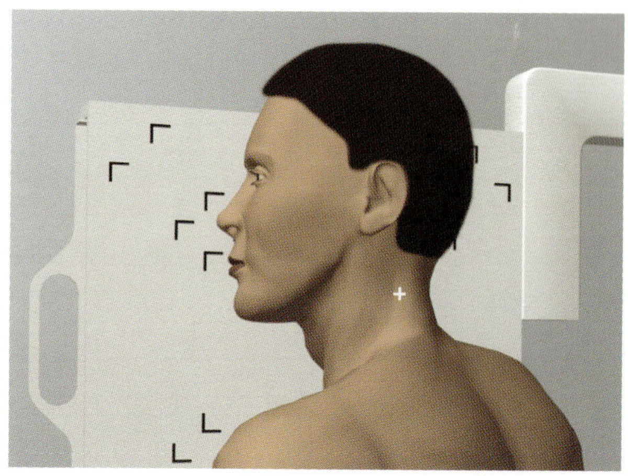

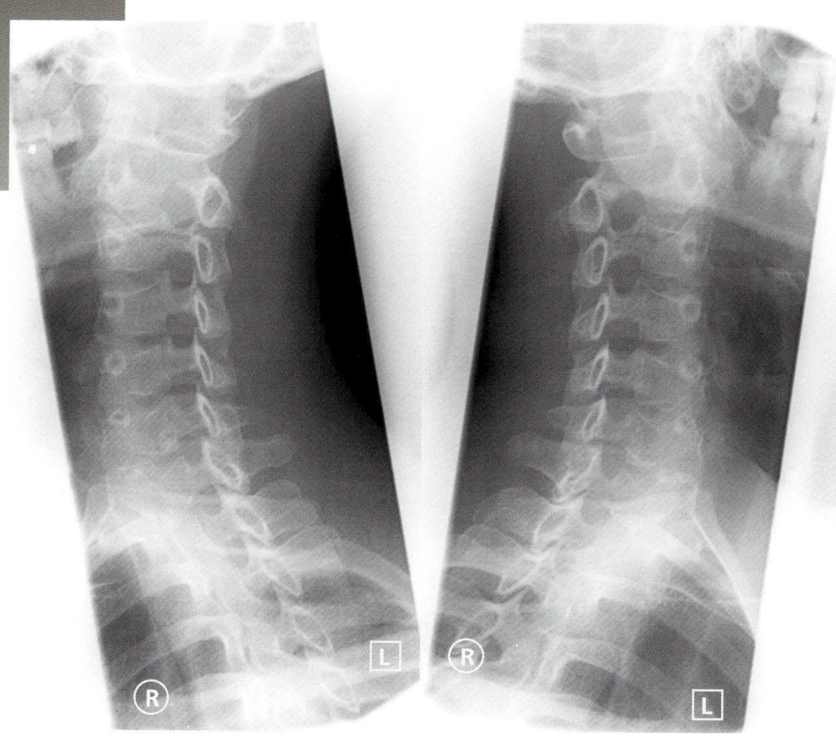

CERVICAL SPINE AP Supine – vertical beam angled 15° as shown ADDITIONAL

Use after injury

Cassette speed

Cassette with screen-film combination, nominal speed 200/400 in the cassette holder

Cassette size

24×30 cm (10×12 inches)
18×24 cm (8×10 inches) for a child
Use a **R**ight or **L**eft marker

Exposure values	mAs	
70 **kV**	"blue" system 200	"green" system 400
Average	25	12.5
Range	20–50	10–25

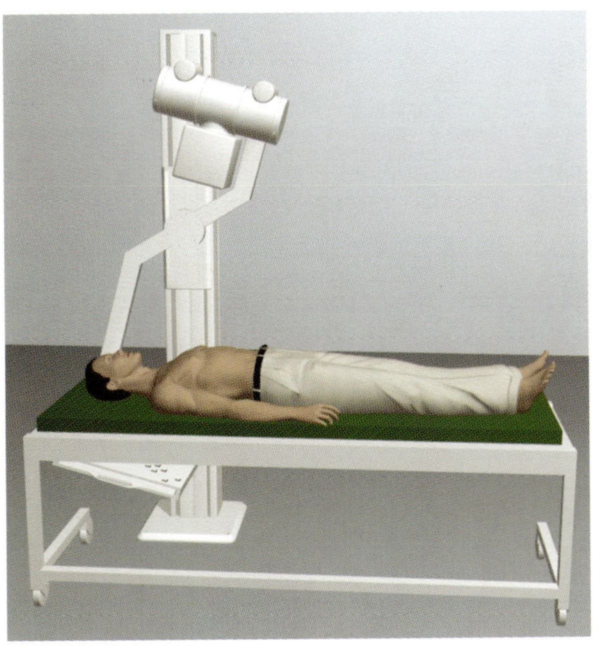

1. Bring in the patient, put the cassette in the cassette holder. Collimate to the format. Angle the tube cassette holder arm.
2. Remove necklace, hairgrips and anything else from the hair.
3. Position the patient. Center and collimate further, if possible. Tell the patient to stop breathing if possible.
4. Expose. Tell the patient to breathe normally.

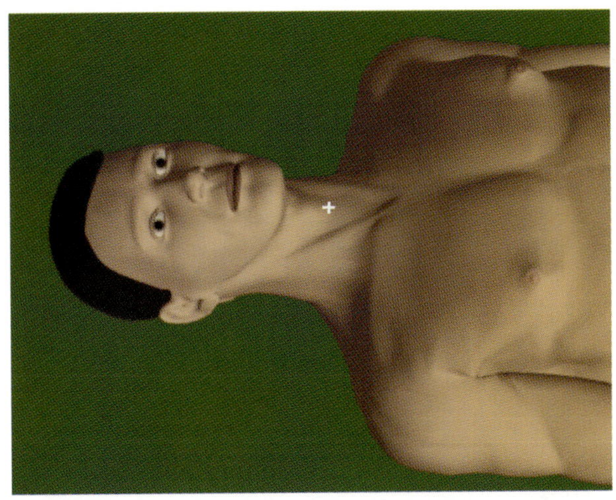

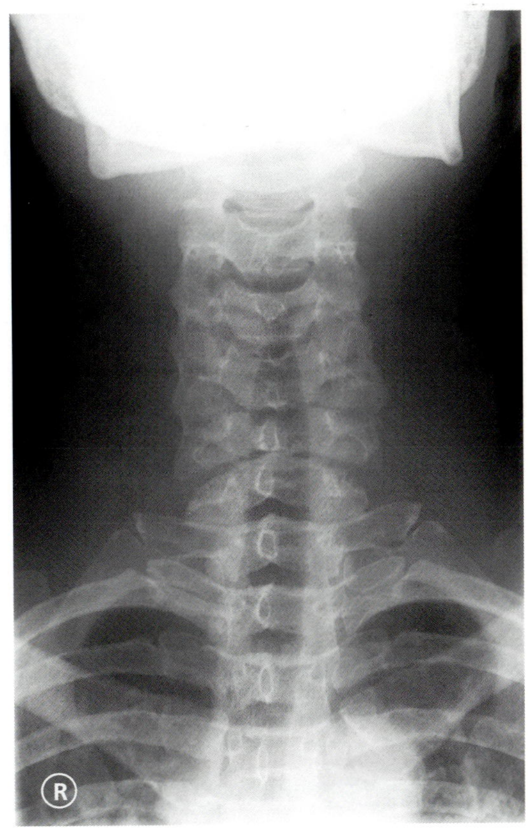

CERVICAL SPINE LATERAL **Supine – horizontal beam** ADDITIONAL

Use after injury

IF A NECK FRACTURE IS SUSPECTED, THE HEAD SHOULD NOT BE LIFTED ONTO A PAD BY THE OPERATOR WITHOUT THE DOCTOR'S PERMISSION.

Cassette speed
Cassette with screen-film combination, nominal speed 200/400 in the cassette holder

Cassette size
24×30 cm (10×12 inches)

Exposure values	mAs	
70 **kV**	"blue" system 200	"green" system 400
Average	25	12.5
Range	16–63	8–32

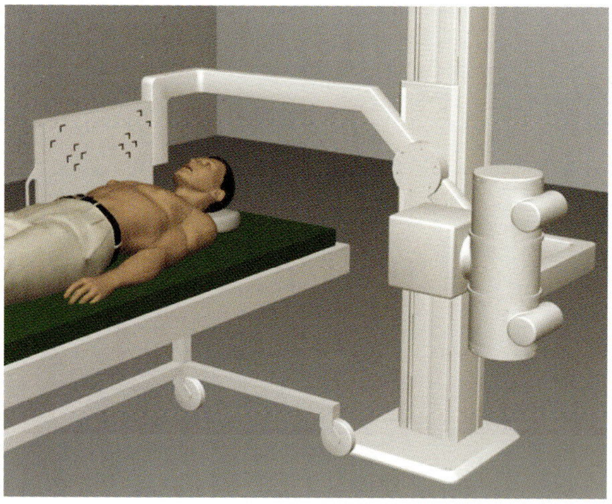

1. Bring in the patient, put the cassette in the cassette holder. Collimate to the format.
2. Remove necklace, hairgrips, earclips and anything else from the hair.
3. The head could be supported by a pad. The head should be in the position, which is the least painful for the patient. If possible, an accompanying person (wearing a lead apron and lead gloves) may pull the arms downwards, to lower the shoulders.
4. Center and collimate further, if possible. Tell the patient to stop breathing.
5. Expose. Tell the patient to breathe normally.

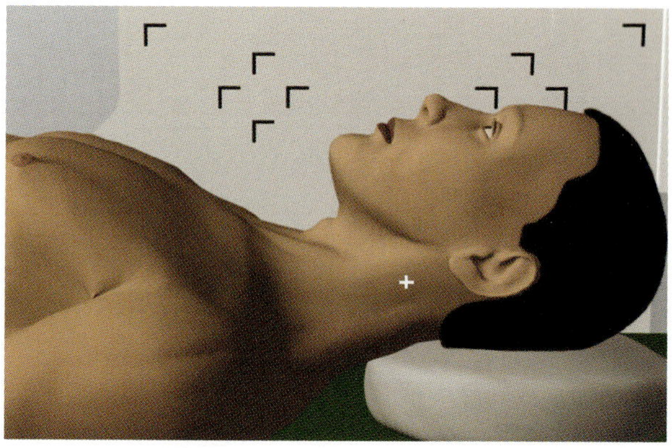

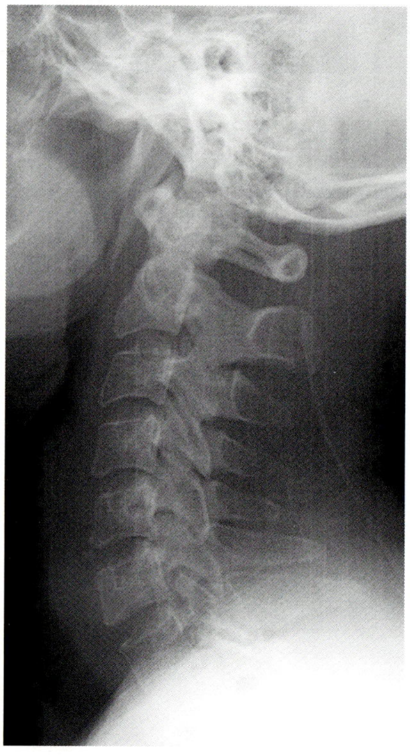

ODONTOID PROCESS AP **Supine – vertical beam angled 10° as shown** ADDITIONAL

First and second cervical vertebrae through the **open mouth**

Cassette speed
Cassette with screen-film combination, nominal speed 200/400 in the cassette holder

Cassette size
18×24 cm (8×10 inches)
Use a **R**ight or **L**eft marker

Exposure values	mAs	
70 **kV**	"blue" system 200	"green" system 400
Average	40	20
Range	20–80	12.5–32

1. Bring in the patient, put the cassette in the cassette holder. Collimate to the format.
2. Remove dentures, hairgrips and anything from the hair.
3. Tell the patient to open the mouth as widely as possible. If the patient is unable to keep the mouth open, place a wedge of soft wood or cork between the upper and lower row of teeth or gums.
4. Center as shown. Collimate further, if possible. Tell the patient to stop breathing.
5. Expose. Tell the patient to breathe normally.
6. Remove the wedge of cork.

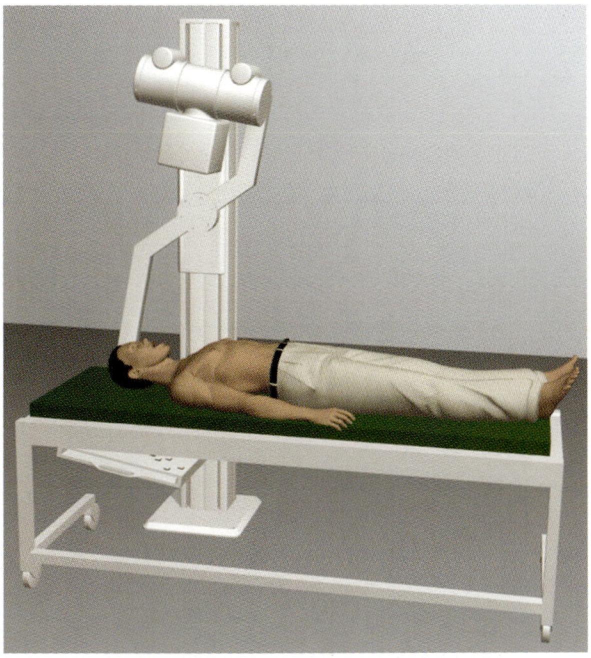

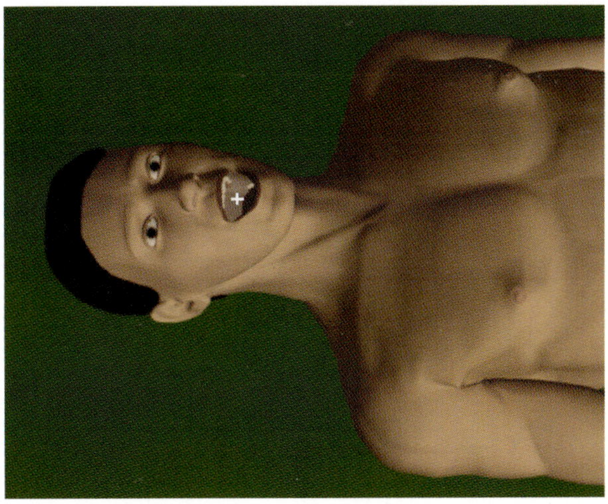

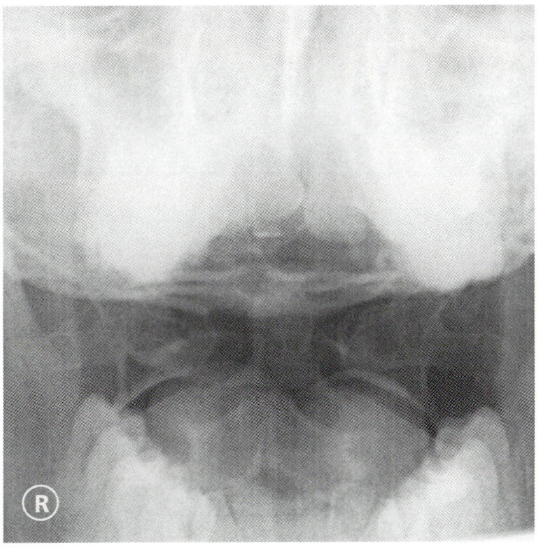

CERVICOTHORACIC REGION LATERAL **Sitting erect** ADDITIONAL

Also possible lying on one side. Seldom needed below the age of 16 years.

Cassette speed
Cassette with screen-film combination, nominal speed 200/400 in the cassette holder

Cassette size
24×30 cm (10×12 inches)

Exposure values	mAs	
80 **kV**	"blue" system 200	"green" system 400/450
Average	100	50
Range	50–160	25–80

1. Bring in the patient, put the cassette in the cassette holder. Collimate to the format.
2. Position the patient with the arm close to the cassette holder elevated following the direction of the cervical spine. The other shoulder should be as low as possible.
3. Center and collimate further, if possible. Tell the patient to stop breathing.
4. Expose. Tell the patient to breathe normally.

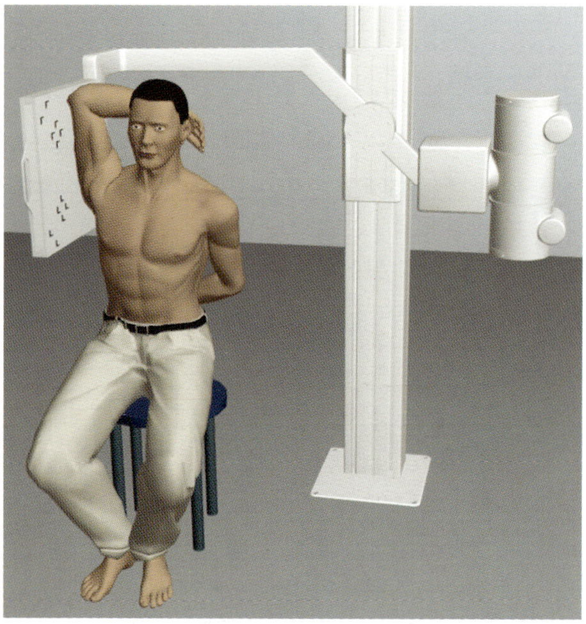

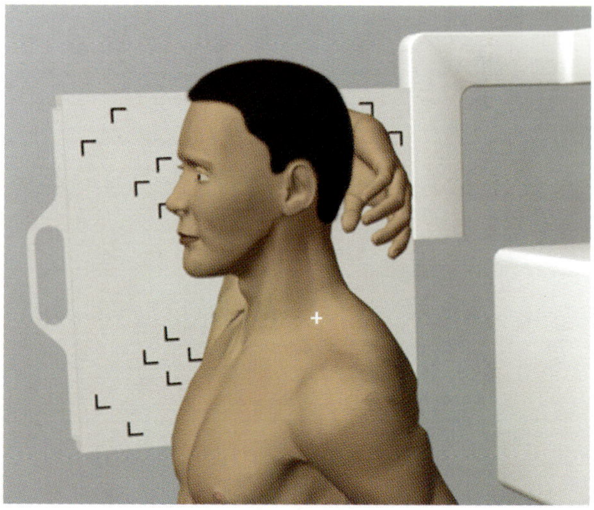

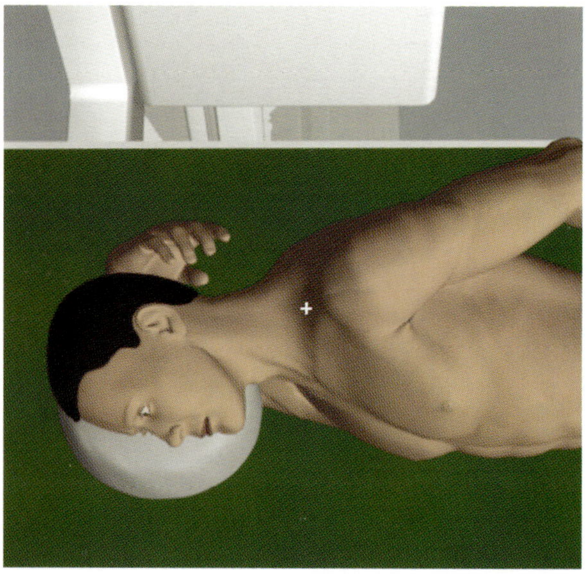

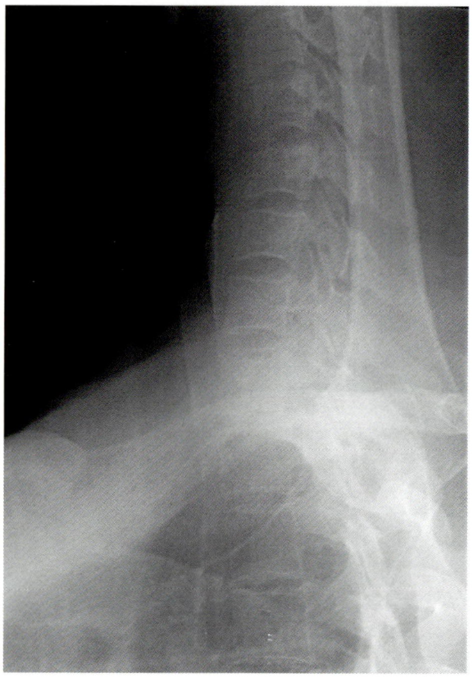

THORACIC SPINE AP **Supine** BASIC

Cassette speed
Cassette with screen-film combination, nominal speed 200/400 in the cassette holder

Cassette size
18×43 cm (7×17 inches)
Use a **R**ight or **L**eft marker

Exposure values	mAs	
70 **kV**	"blue" system 200	"green" system 400
Average	80	40
Range	63–200	32–100

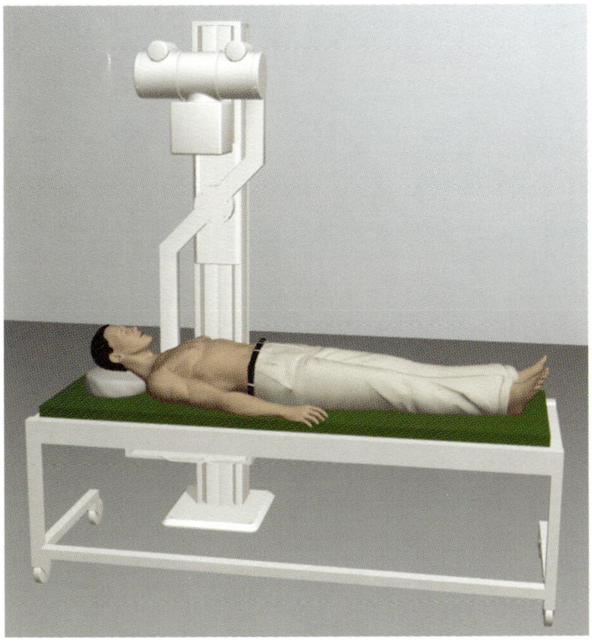

1. Bring in the patient, put the cassette in the cassette holder. Collimate to the format.
2. Position the patient.
3. Center and collimate further, if possible. Tell the patient to stop breathing.
4. Expose. Tell the patient to breathe normally.

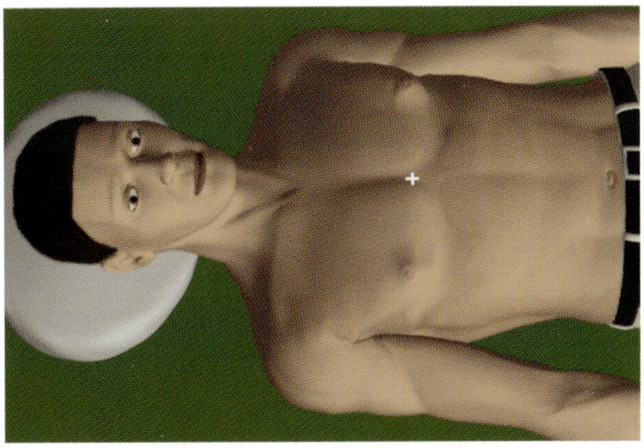

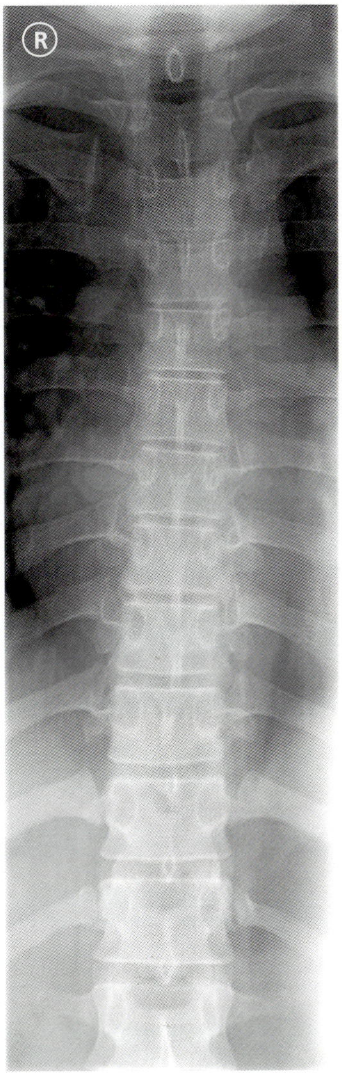

THORACIC SPINE LATERAL Lying on the left (or right side) BASIC

Cassette speed
Cassette with screen-film combination, nominal speed 200/400 in the cassette holder

Cassette size
18×43 cm (7×17 inches) or 20×40 cm

Exposure values	mAs	
70 **kV**	"blue" system 200	"green" system 400
Average	160	80
Range	40–200	32–160

1. Bring in the patient, put the cassette in the cassette holder. Collimate to the format.
2. Position the patient. Bend the knees to stabilize the body. The long axis of the spine should be horizontal.
4. Center and collimate further, if possible.
3. Expose while the patient is breathing as usual.

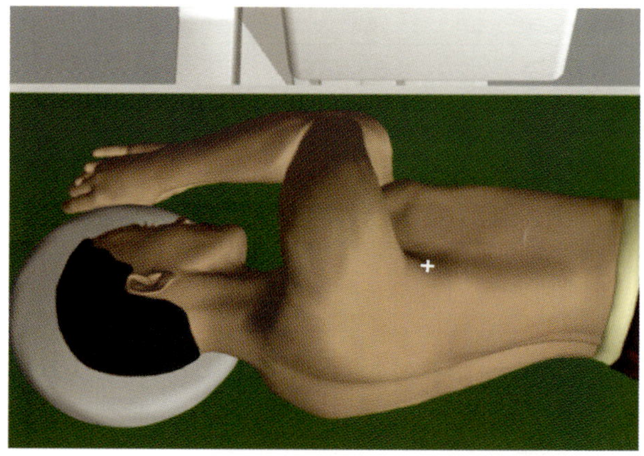

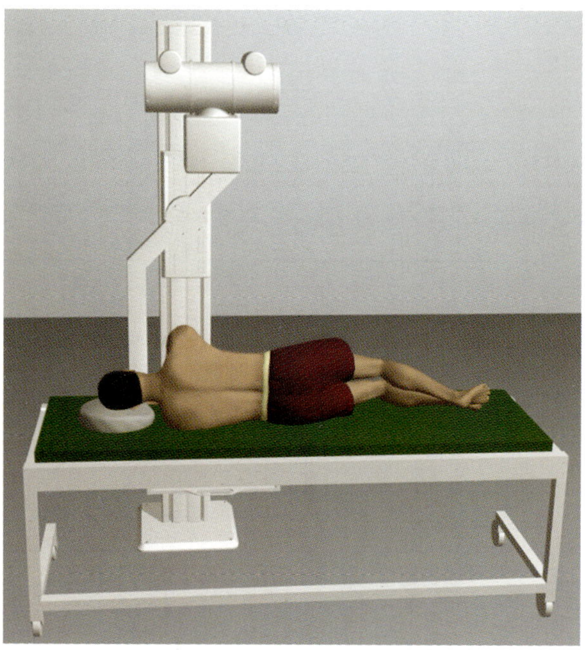

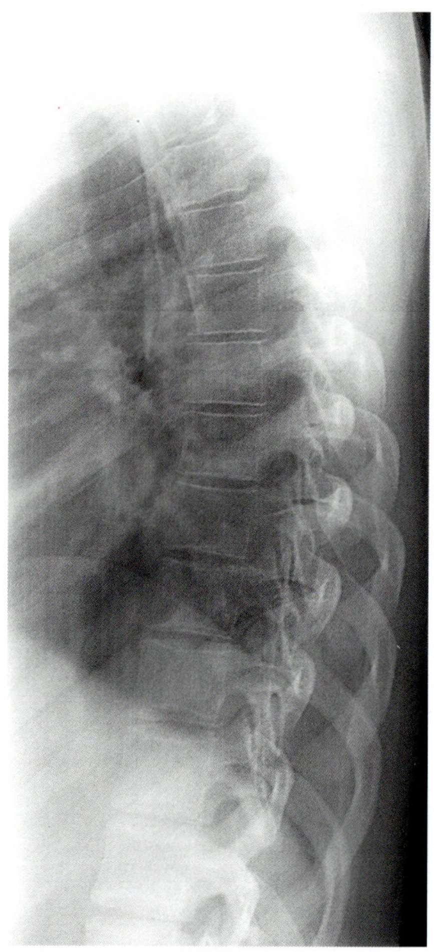

LUMBAR SPINE AP (or PA) Supine (or prone) BASIC

AFTER INJURY—DO NOT TURN THE PATIENT OVER. X-RAY IN EITHER AP OR PA POSITION WITH AS LITTLE MOVEMENT AS POSSIBLE.

Cassette speed
Cassette with screen-film combination, nominal speed 200/400 in the cassette holder

Cassette size
18×43 cm (7×17 inches)
Use a **R**ight or **L**eft marker

Exposure values	mAs	
70 **kV**	"blue" system 200	"green" system 400
Average	100	50
Range	50–160	25–80

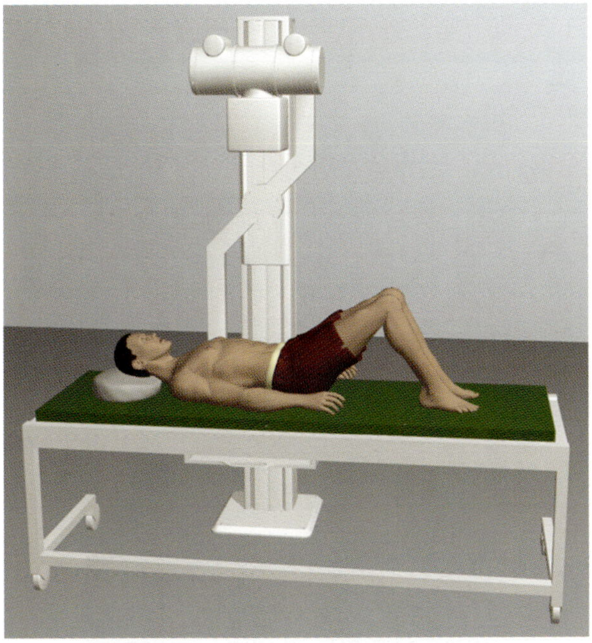

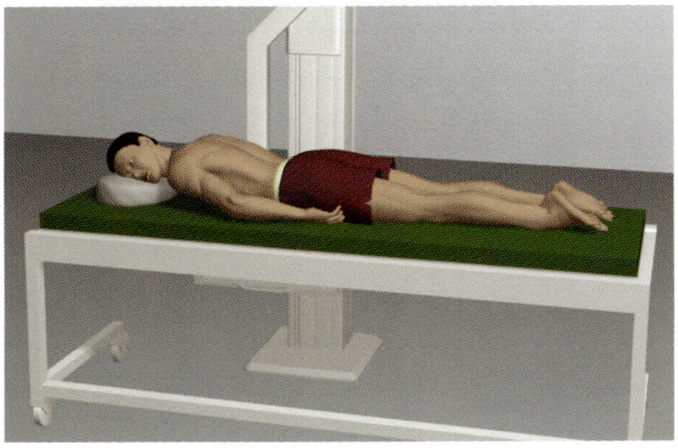

1. Bring in the patient, put the cassette in the cassette holder. Collimate to the format.
2. Position the patient. THE PATIENT'S KNEES SHOULD BE BENT SO THAT THE PATIENT'S BACK IS FLAT ON THE TABLE.
3. Center and collimate further, if possible. Tell the patient to stop breathing.
4. Expose. Tell the patient to breathe normally.

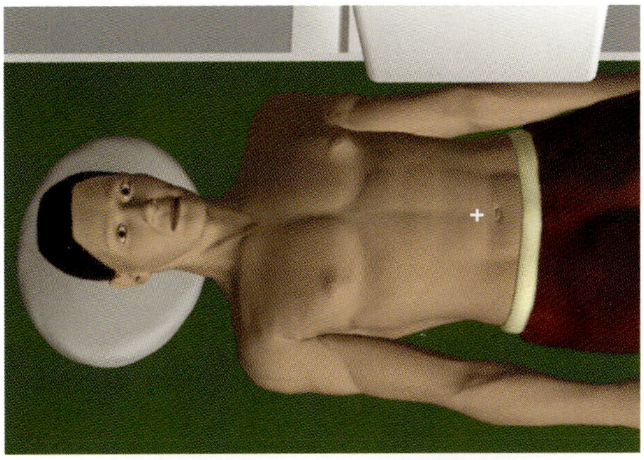

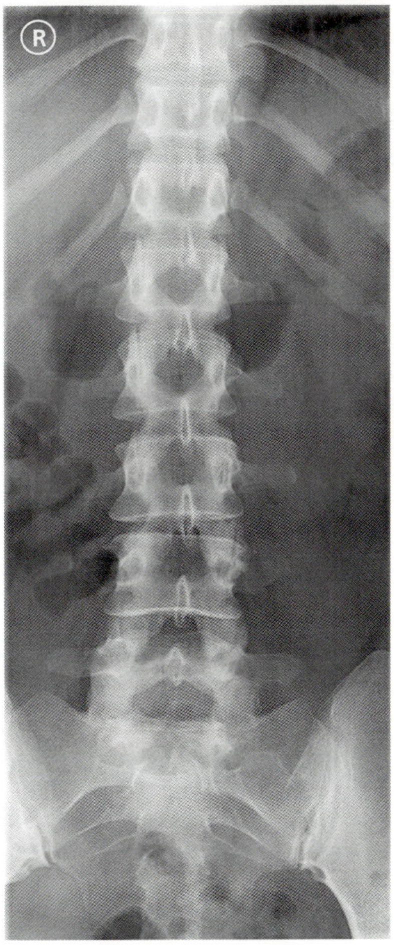

LUMBAR SPINE LATERAL Lying on the left (or right) side BASIC

If a fracture is suspected, use SPINE 12

Cassette speed

Cassette with screen-film combination, nominal speed 200/400 in the cassette holder

Cassette size

18×43 cm (7×17 inches) or 20×40 cm

Exposure values	mAs average (range)	
kV	"blue" system 200	"green" system 400/450/500
80	–	100 (50–200)
90	160 (100–250)	(160–250)
120	(125–250)	–

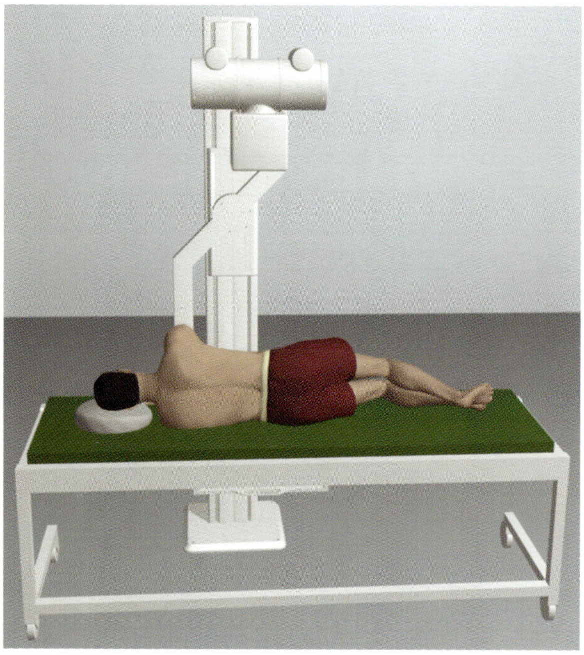

1. Bring in the patient, put the cassette in the cassette holder. Collimate to the format.
2. Position the patient. Bend the knees to stabilize the body. Center and collimate further, if possible.
3. Tell the patient to breath in, then out, and then stop breathing. Expose.
4. Tell the patient to breathe normally.

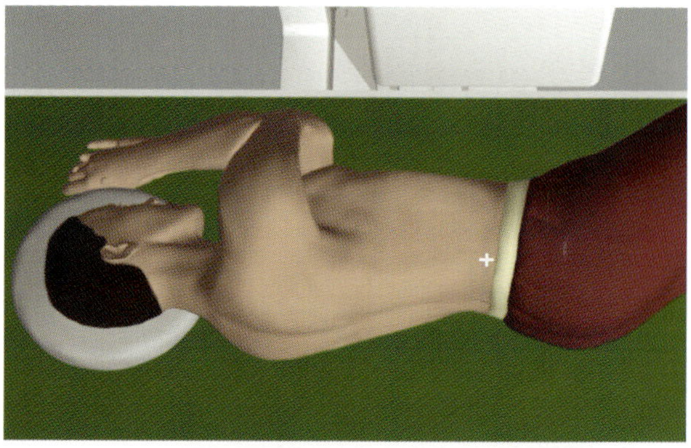

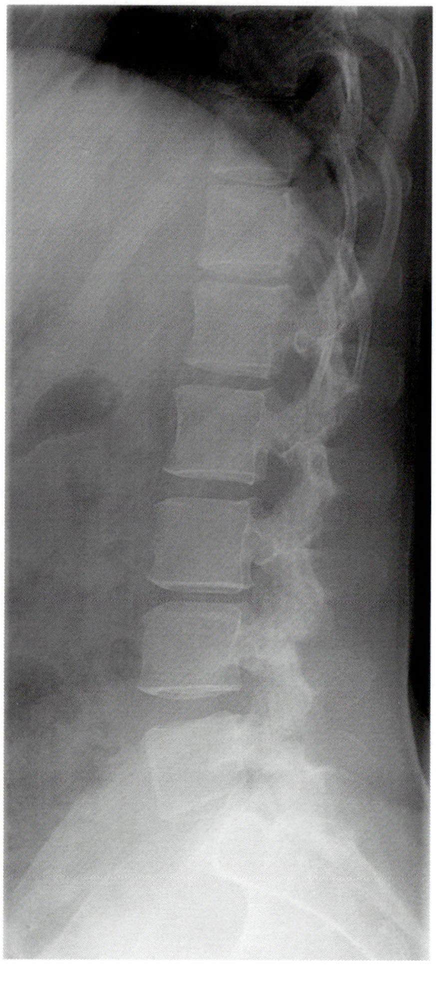

LUMBAR SPINE LATERAL – after injury   Supine – horizontal beam   ADDITIONAL

Cassette speed
Cassette with screen-film combination, nominal speed 200/400 in the cassette holder

Cassette size
18×43 cm (7×17 inches) or 20×40 cm

Exposure values	mAs average (range)	
kV	"blue" system 200	"green" system 400/450/500
80	–	100 (50–200)
90	160 (100–250)	(160–250)
120	(125–250)	–

1. Bring in the patient, put the cassette in the cassette holder. Collimate to the format.
2. Position the patient. Center and collimate further, if possible. Tell the patient to stop breathing.
3. Expose. Tell the patient to breathe normally.

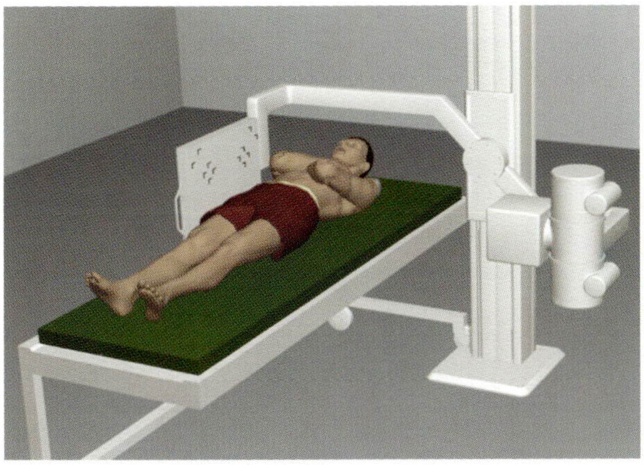

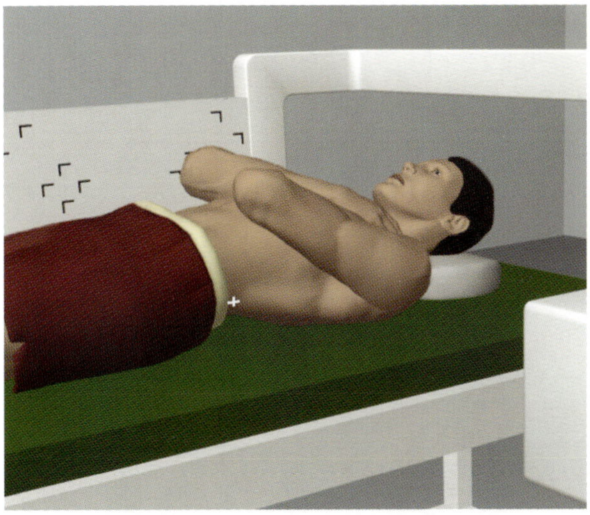

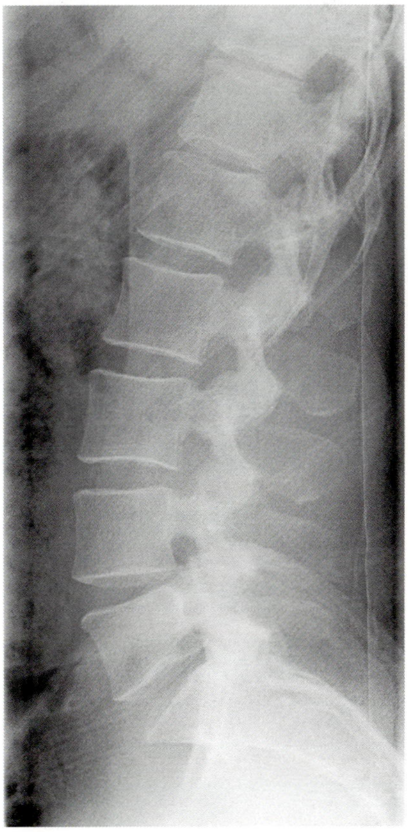

SACRUM AP: Lumbosacral junction and sacroiliac joints

Supine – vertical beam angled 15° as shown BASIC

Do not use for children

Cassette speed

Cassette with screen-film combination, nominal speed 200/400 in the cassette holder

Cassette size

24×30 cm (10×12 inches)

Use a **R**ight or **L**eft marker

Exposure values	mAs	
70 **kV**	"blue" system 200	"green" system 400
Average	125	63
Range	80–250	40–125

1. Bring in the patient, put the cassette in the cassette holder. Collimate to the format.
2. Angle the tube cassette holder arm.
3. Position the patient. Center 3 cm above the symphysis and collimate further, if possible.
4. Expose while the patient is breathing as usual.

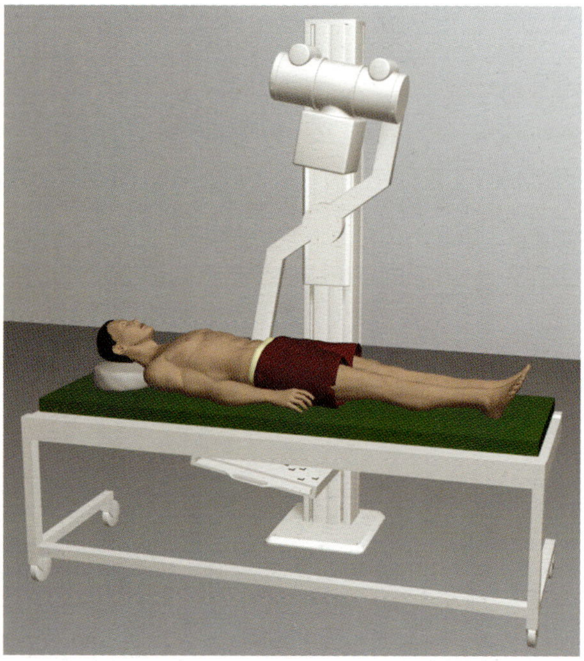

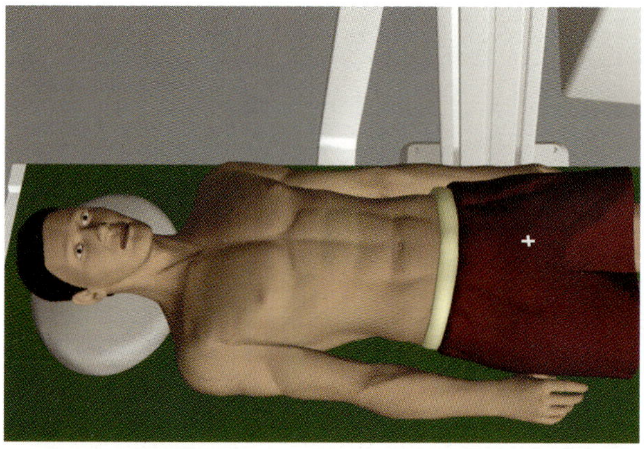

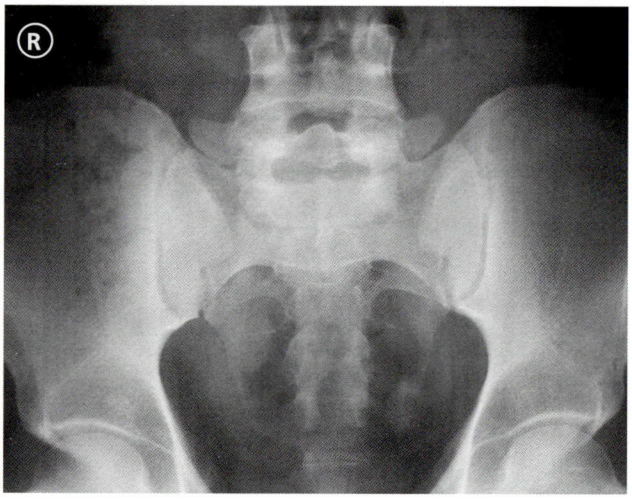

LUMBOSACRAL JUNCTION LATERAL   Lying on the left (or right) side   BASIC

Do not use for children

Cassette speed
Cassette with screen-film combination, nominal speed 200/400 in the cassette holder

Cassette size
24×30 cm (10×12 inches)

Exposure values	mAs average (range)	
kV	"blue" system 200	"green" system 400/500
90	(100–250)	125 (50–250)
120	125 (125–250)	(125–160)

1. Bring in the patient, put the cassette in the cassette holder. Collimate to the format.
2. Position the patient. Bend the knees to stabilize the body. Support with a pad under the waist. Center 3 cm below the iliac crest and collimate further, if possible.
3. Tell the patient to stop breathing. Expose.
4. Tell the patient to breathe normally.

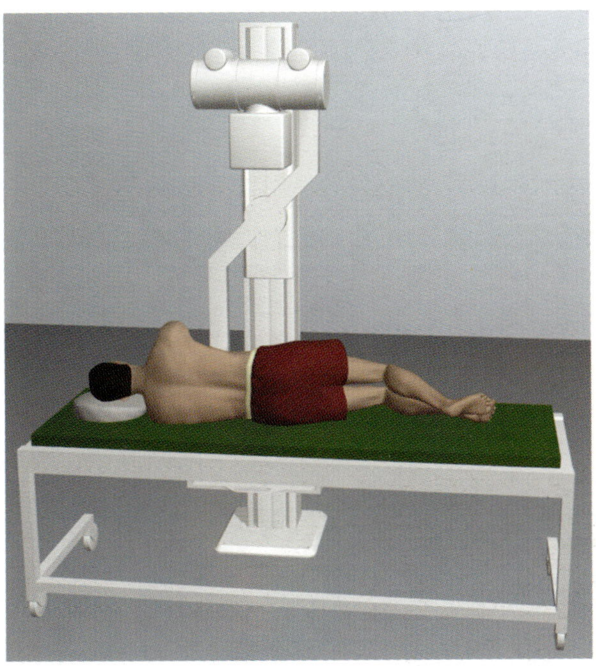

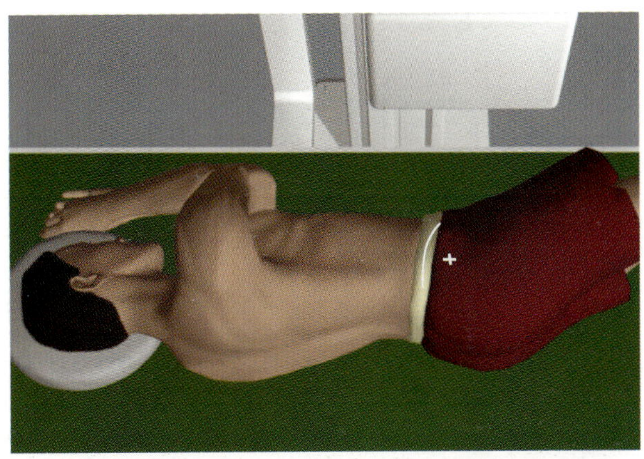

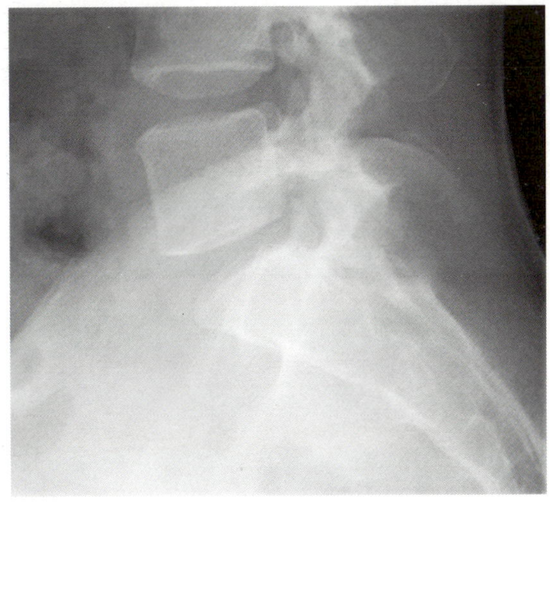

Arm

CLAVICLE

1. Clavicle AP – two angled views, page 62.

SCAPULA

2. Scapula AP, page 63.
3. Scapula lateral, page 64.

SHOULDER JOINT

X-rays of the shoulder joint are taken with the patient lying down, unless there is pain.

4. Shoulder AP – two views taken with different rotation of the arm, page 65.
5. Shoulder AP – acromioclavicular joint, page 66.
6 Shoulder axial, page 67.

Patient with the arm in pain (after injury)

7. Shoulder AP, page 68.
8. Shoulder lateral, page 69.

HUMERUS

X-rays of the humerus are taken with the patient lying down, unless there is pain

9. Humerus AP and lateral – two views taken with different rotation of the arm, page 70.

Patient with the arm in pain (after injury)

10. Humerus AP, page 71.
11. Humerus lateral, page 72.

ELBOW

12. Elbow AP, page 73.
13. Elbow lateral, page 74.
14. Elbow semiflexed – after injury, two views to be taken, page 75.

FOREARM

15. Forearm PA – after injury, page 76.
16. Forearm lateral – after injury, page 77.

WRIST

17. Wrist PA and additional view in ulnar deviation, page 78.
18. Wrist lateral, page 79.
19. Scaphoid – after injury, page 80.

HAND

20. Hand PA and additional two oblique views, page 81.
21. Thumb AP, page 82.
22. Thumb lateral, page 83.
23. Single finger lateral, page 84.

CLAVICLE AP Supine – vertical beam angulated +20° and –20° as shown BASIC

Two views

Cassette speed
Cassette with screen-film combination, nominal speed 200/400 in the cassette holder
For a CHILD, cassette **on** the table

Cassette size
24×30 cm (10×12 inches)
18×24 cm (8×10 inches) for a child
Use a **R**ight or **L**eft marker

Exposure values	mAs	
70 **kV**	"blue" system 200	"green" system 400
Average	25	12.5
Range	20–50	10–25
Child 53 **kV**	"blue" system 200	"green" system 400/250
Average	6.3	5

1. Bring in the patient, put the cassette in the cassette holder or on the table (for a child). Collimate to the format.
2. Angle the tube cassette holder arm.
3. Position the patient. Center and collimate further, if possible.
4. Expose.
5. Change cassette and angle, expose again.

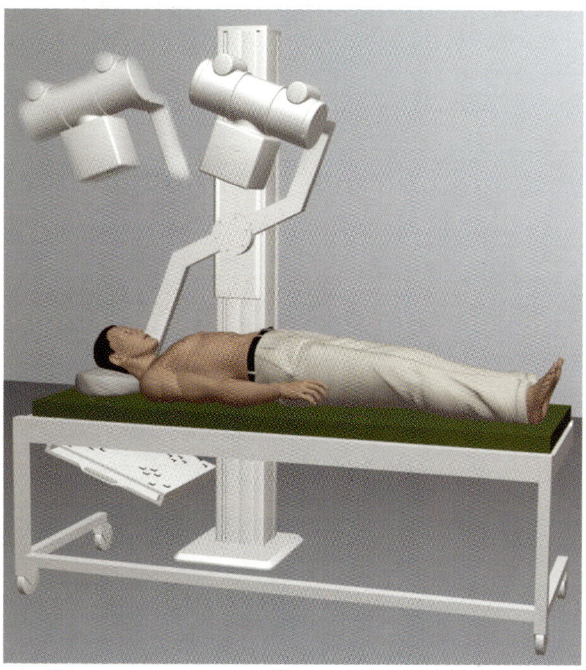

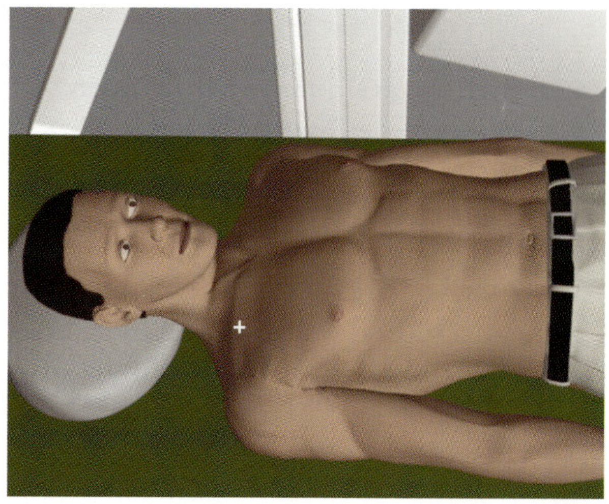

Center point: mid clavicle

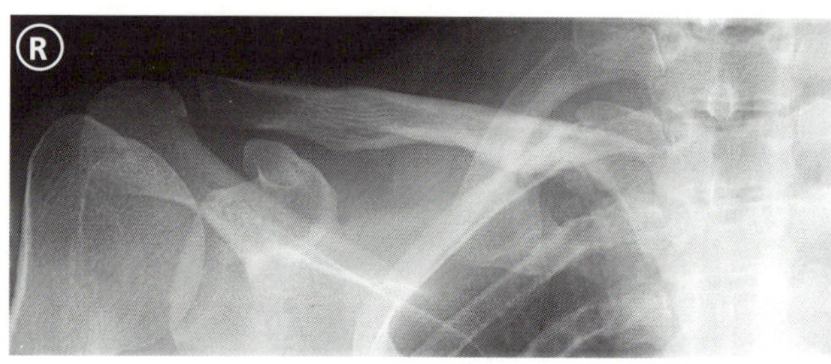

X-ray with angulation as shown

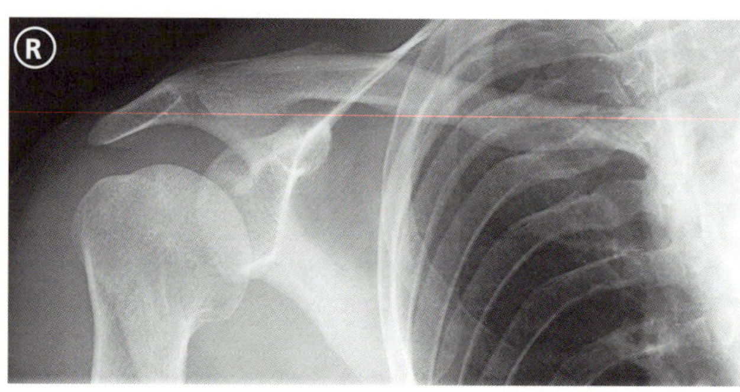

X-ray with the opposite angulation

SCAPULA AP **Supine** BASIC

If the patient is in pain, use ARM 7

Cassette speed
Cassette with screen-film combination, nominal speed 200/400 in the cassette holder
For a CHILD, cassette **on** the table

Cassette size
24×30 cm (10×12 inches)
18×24 cm (8×10 inches) for a child
Use a **R**ight or **L**eft marker

Exposure values	mAs	
70 **kV**	"blue" system 200	"green" system 400
Average	25	12.5
Range	20–50	10–25
Child 53 **kV**	"blue" system 200	"green" system 400/250
Average	6.3	5

1. Bring in the patient, put the cassette in the cassette holder. Collimate to the format.
2. Position the patient. Use a pillow under the other shoulder. Center and collimate further, if possible.
3. Expose.

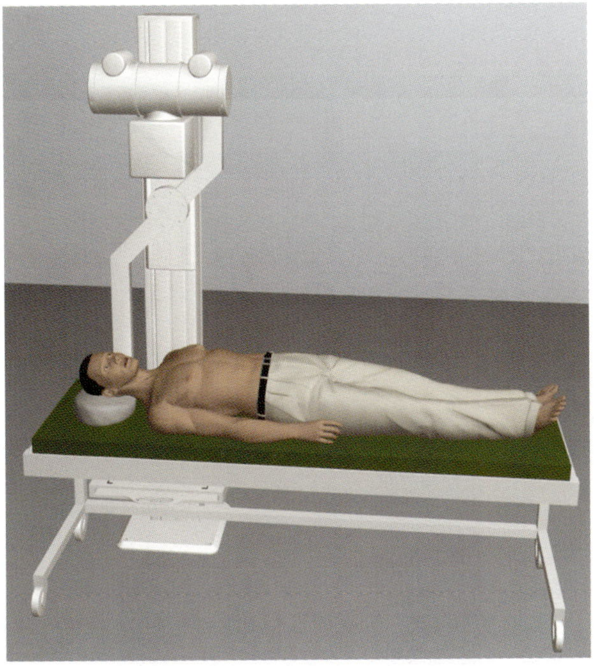

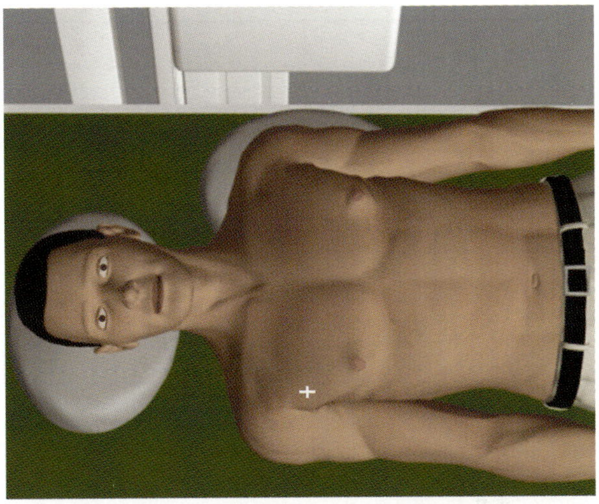

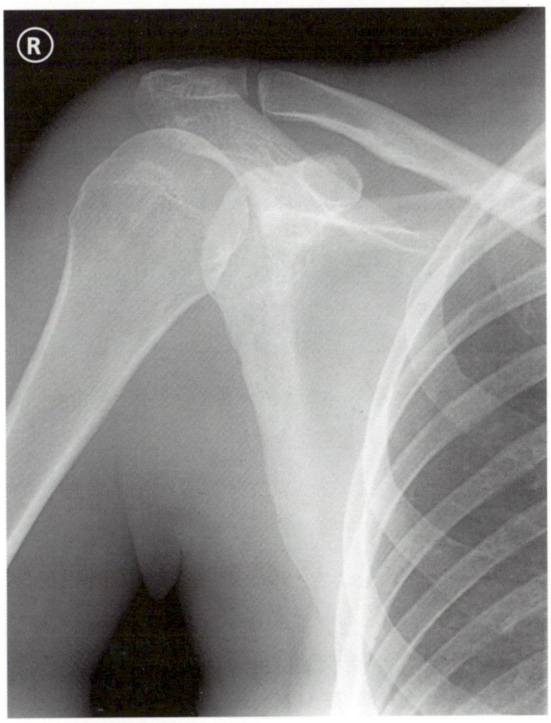

SCAPULA LATERAL Sitting erect BASIC

Do not use for children under 10 years of age

Cassette speed
Cassette with screen-film combination, nominal speed 200/400 in the cassette holder

Cassette size
24×30 cm (10×12 inches)
Use a **R**ight or **L**eft marker

Exposure values	mAs	
70 **kV**	"blue" system 200	"green" system 400
Average	50	25
Range	40–125	20–64

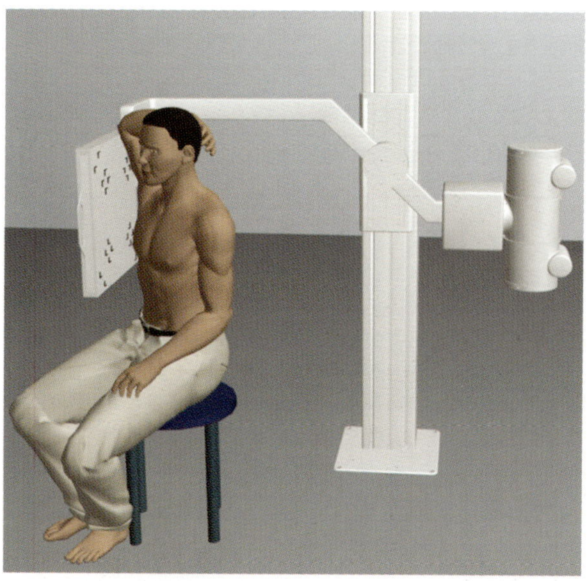

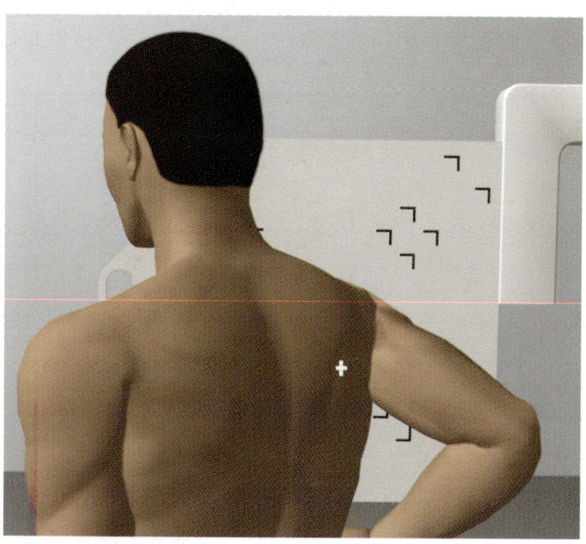

Alternative position

1. Bring in the patient, put the cassette in the cassette holder. Collimate to the format.
2. Position the patient. Unless the patient is in pain raise the arm with the hand behind the head. See alternative position with the arm down, when it is painful. Center and collimate further, if possible.
3. Expose.

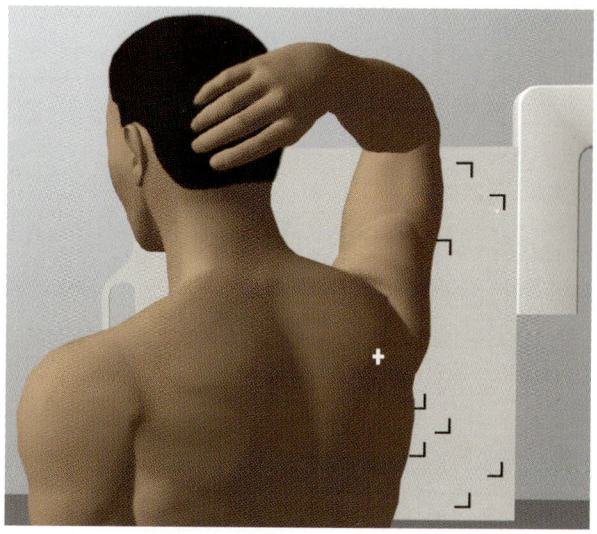

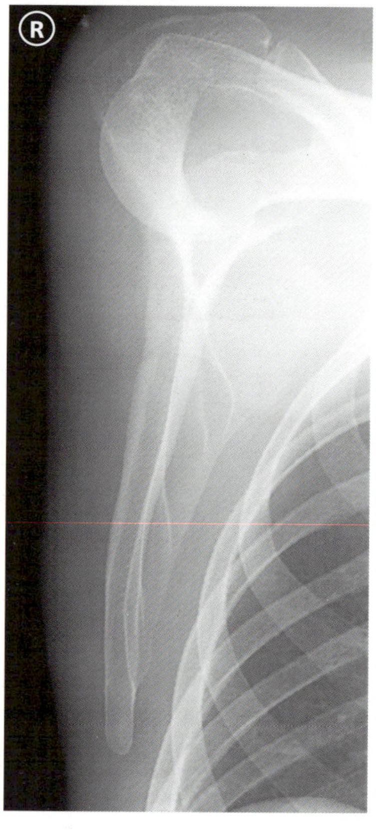

SHOULDER AP – two views Supine – vertical beam angled 10° as shown BASIC

Cassette speed
Cassette with screen-film combination, nominal speed 200/400 in the cassette holder
For a CHILD, cassette **on** the table (one view)

Cassette size
24×30 cm (10×12 inches)
18×24 cm (8×10 inches) for a child
Use a **R**ight or **L**eft marker

Exposure values	mAs	
70 **kV**	"blue" system 200	"green" system 400
Average	12.5	6.3
Range	10–25	5–12.5
Child 53 **kV**	"blue" system 200	"green" system 400/250
Average	4	3.2

1. Bring in the patient, put the cassette in the cassette holder or on the table (for a child). Collimate to the format.
2. Position the patient.
   a. Place a large pillow under the shoulder not to be examined.
   b. Turn the patient so that the shoulder to be X-rayed lies flat on the table.
   c. Rotate the arm outwards so that the palm of the hand faces upwards.
3. Center and collimate further, if possible.
4. Expose and change cassette.
5. Rotate the arm inwards so that the palm of the hand faces downwards. Expose

INFANTS and SMALL CHILDREN lie supine on the cassette on top of the table. Either view only.

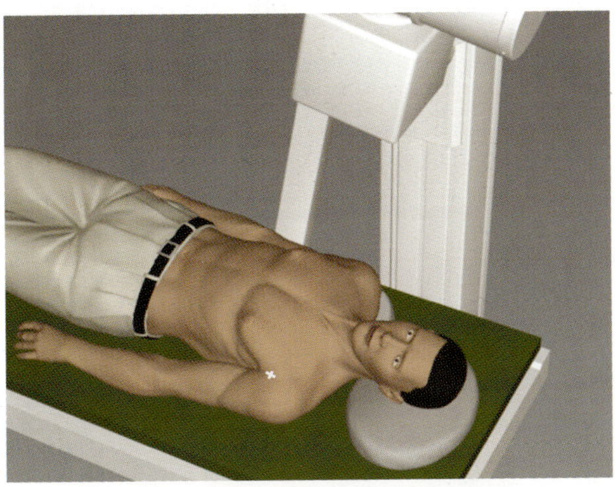

Palm of hand facing down

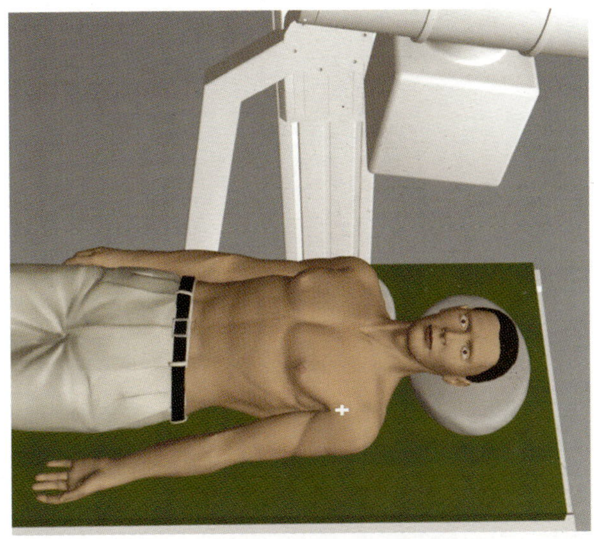

Palm of hand facing up

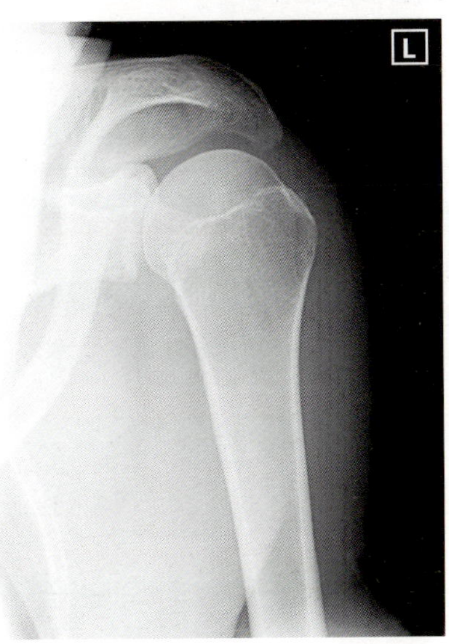

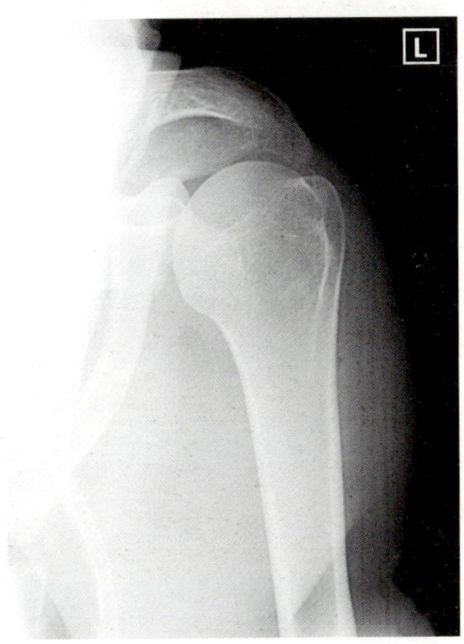

SHOULDER AP Supine ADDITIONAL

Upper arm away from body—acromioclavicular joint

Cassette speed

Cassette with screen-film combination, nominal speed 200/400 in the cassette holder
For a CHILD, cassette **on** the table (one view)

Cassette size

18×24 cm (8×10 inches)
Use a **R**ight or **L**eft marker

Exposure values	mAs (average)	
kV	"blue" system 200	"green" system 400/250
Adult 70	12.5	6.3
Child 53	4	3.2

1. Bring in the patient, put the cassette in the cassette holder or on the table (for a child). Collimate to the format.
2. Position the patient. Bend the upper arm away from body.
3. Center and collimate further, if possible.
4. Expose.

INFANTS and SMALL CHILDREN lie supine on the cassette on top of the table.

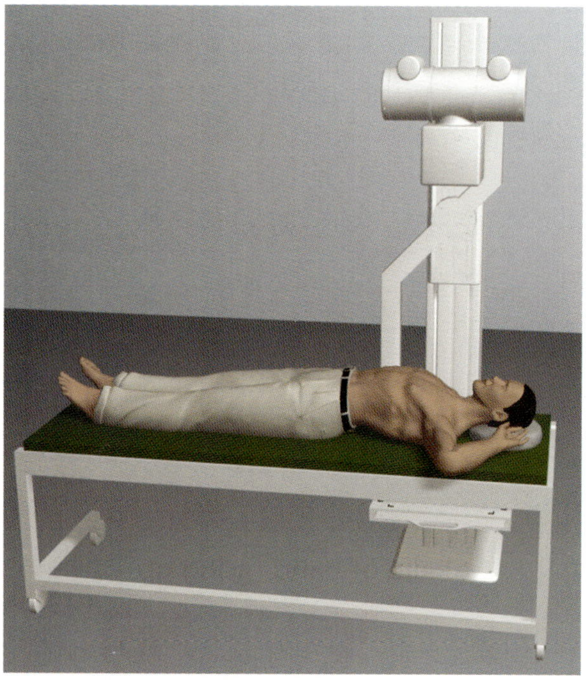

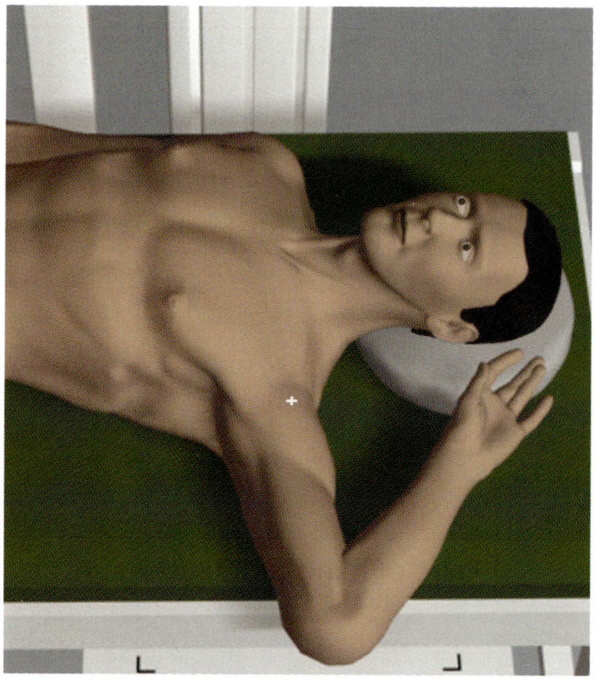

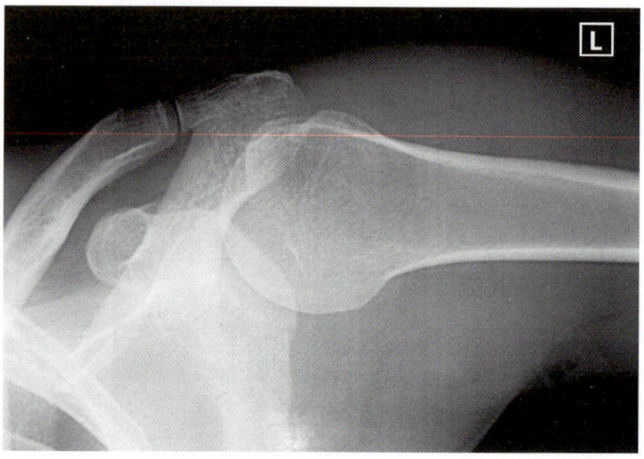

SHOULDER AXIAL ADDITIONAL

Cassette speed
Cassette with screen-film combination, nominal speed 100/200 on top of a firm support (12–15 cm high) on the cassette holder.

Cassette size
18×24 cm (8×10 inches)
Use a **R**ight or **L**eft marker

Exposure values	mAs	
53 **kV**	"blue" system 200	"green" system 100/63
Average	10	25

1. Bring in the patient, put the cassette on top of a firm support (12–15 cm high) on the cassette holder. Collimate to the format.
2. Position the patient. Bend the upper arm away from body.
3. Center and collimate further, if possible.
4. Expose.

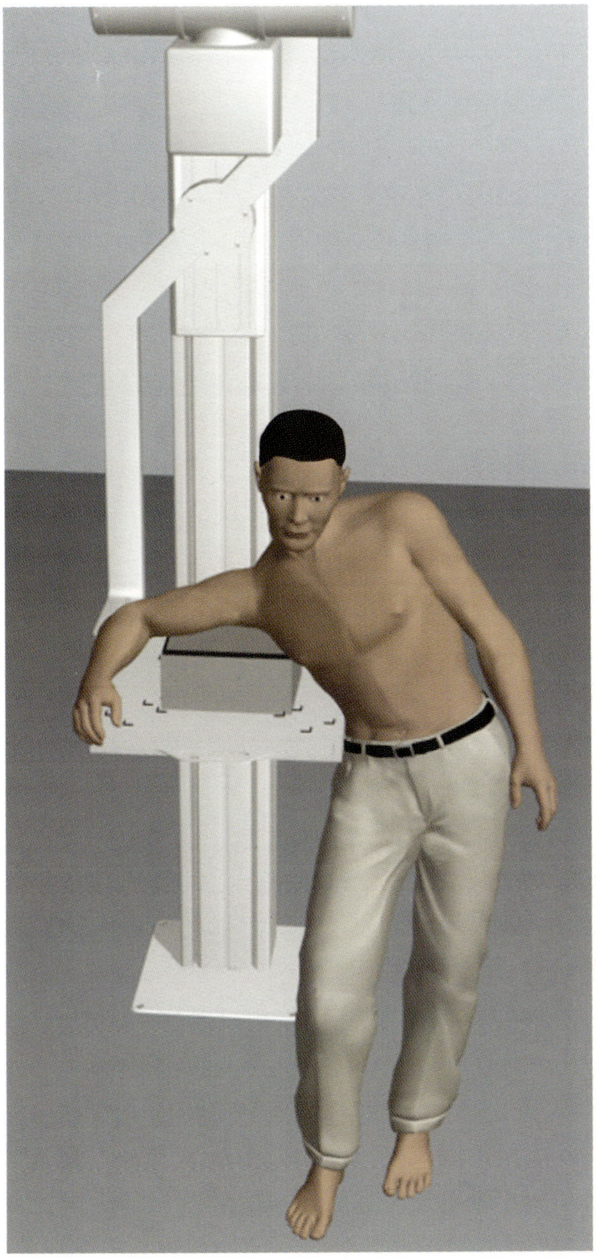

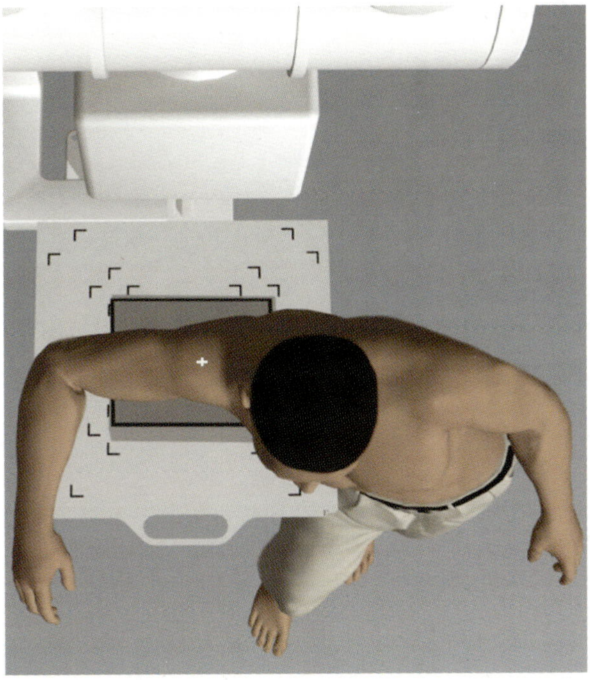

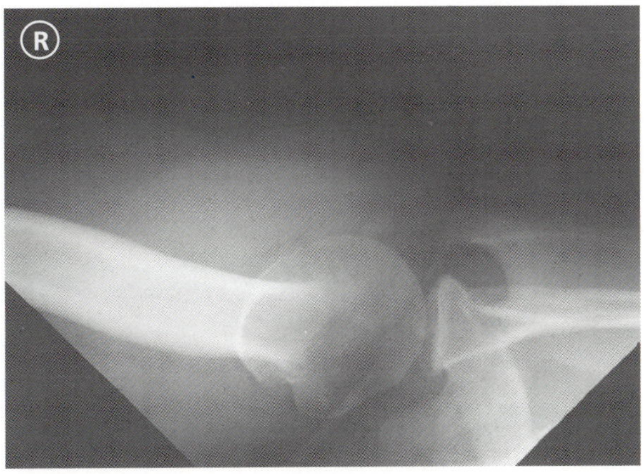

SHOULDER AP Sitting erect ADDITIONAL

After injury

Cassette speed
Cassette with screen-film combination, nominal speed 200/400 in the cassette holder

Cassette size
24×30 cm (10×12 inches)
Use a **R**ight or **L**eft marker

Exposure values	mAs	
70 **kV**	"blue" system 200	"green" system 400
Average	12.5	6.3
Range	10–32	5–16

1. Bring in the patient, put the cassette in the cassette holder. Collimate to the format.
2. Position the patient. The patients forearm should be at right angles to the cassette holder, pointing straight towards the x-ray tube.
3. Center and collimate further, if possible.
4. Expose.

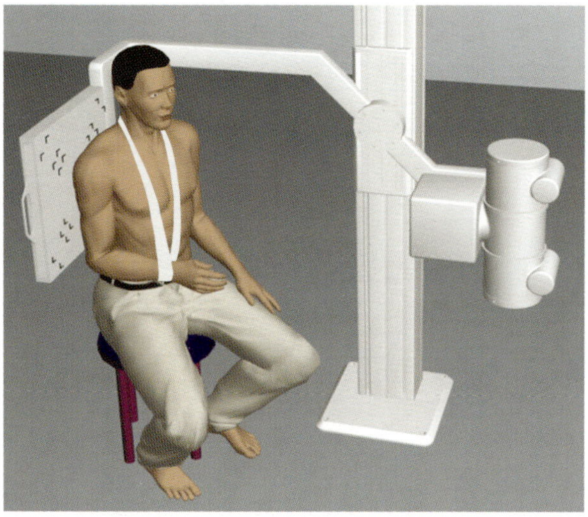

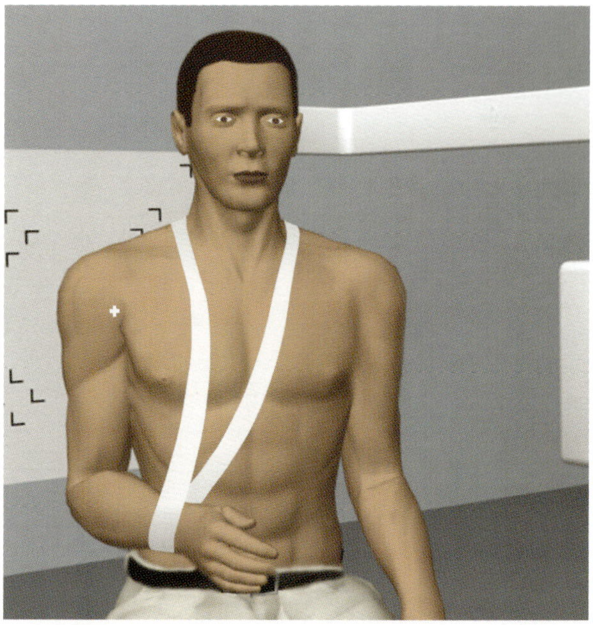

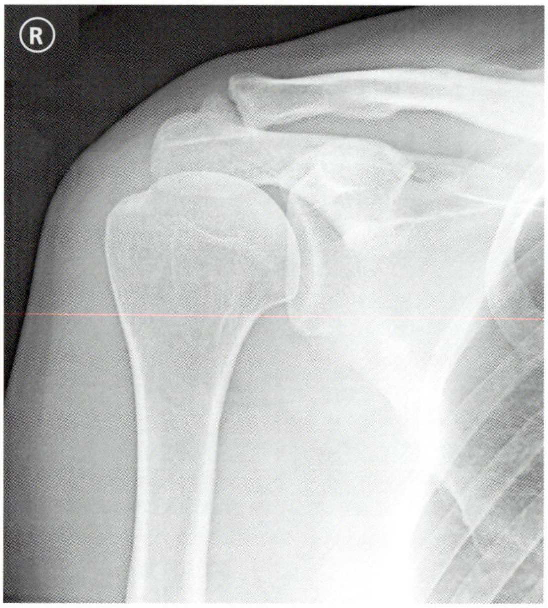

SHOULDER LATERAL – after injury   Sitting erect   ADDITIONAL

Cassette speed
Cassette with screen-film combination, nominal speed 200/400 in the cassette holder

Cassette size
24×30 cm (10×12 inches)
Use a **R**ight or **L**eft marker

Exposure values	mAs	
70 **kV**	"blue" system 200	"green" system 400
Average	32	16
Range	20–50	10–25

1. Bring in the patient, put the cassette in the cassette holder. Collimate to the format.
2. Position the patient. The patients forearm should be close to the cassette holder.
3. Center and collimate further, if possible.
4. Expose.

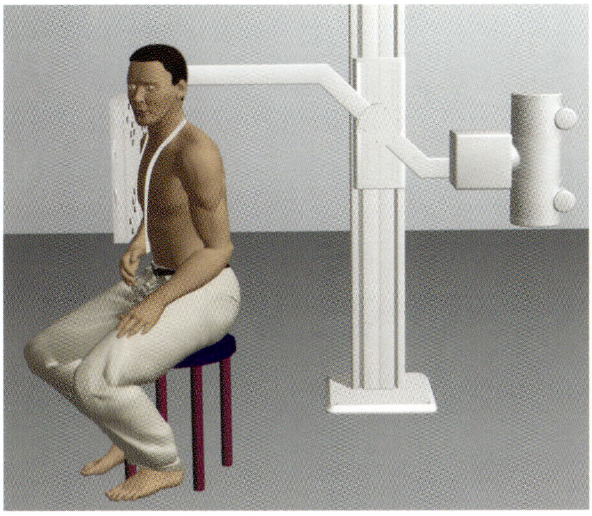

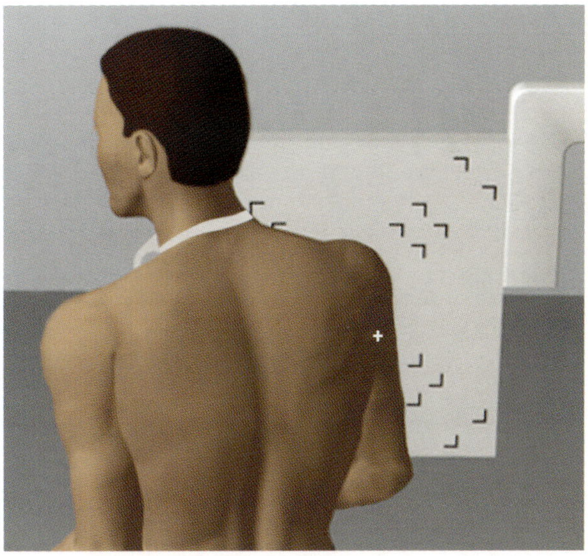

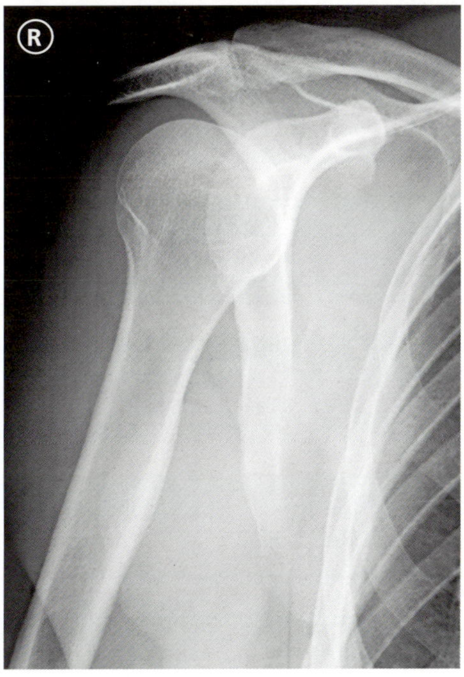

HUMERUS AP and LATERAL – no injury Supine BASIC

Two views

Cassette speed

Cassette with screen-film combination, nominal speed 200/400 on the table

Cassette size

18×43 cm (7×17 inches) or 20×40 cm

Use a **R**ight or **L**eft marker

Exposure values	mAs	
70 **kV**	"blue" system 200	"green" system 400
Average	12.5	6.3
Range	8–16	4–8

1. Bring in the patient, put the cassette on the table. Collimate to the format.
2. Position the patient. Rotate the arm outwards so that the palm of the hand faces upwards.
3. Center and collimate further, if possible.
4. Expose
6. Change cassette.
7. Rotate the arm inwards so that the palm of the hand faces downwards.
8. Expose.

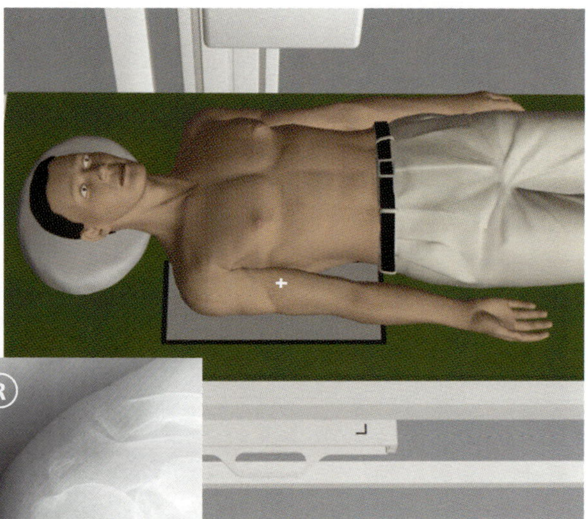

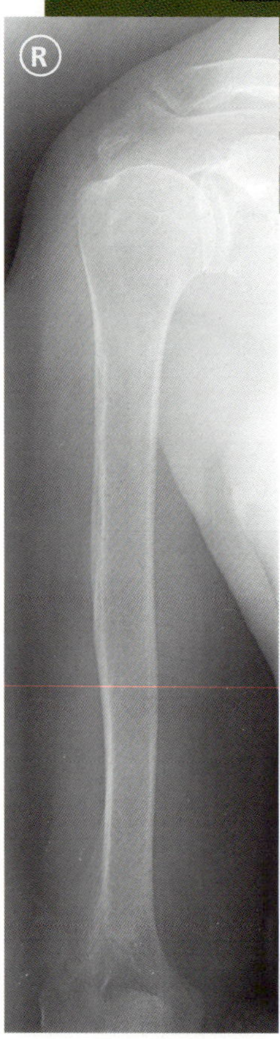

Palm of hand facing up

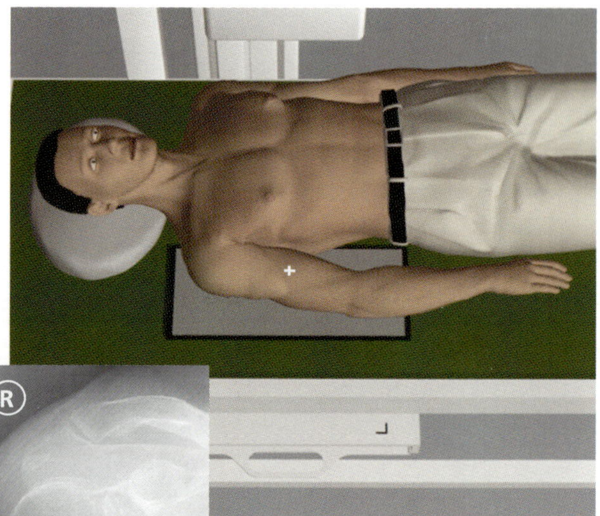

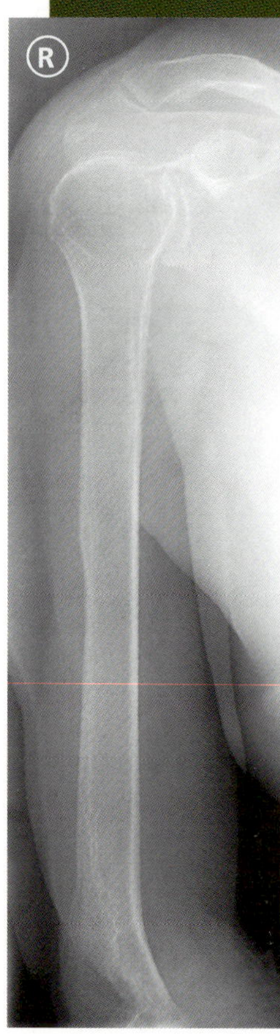

Palm of hand facing down

HUMERUS AP – after injury Sitting erect ADDITIONAL

Cassette speed
Cassette with screen-film combination, nominal speed 200/400 in the cassette holder

Cassette size
18×43 cm (7×17 inches) or 20×40 cm
Use a **R**ight or **L**eft marker

Exposure values	mAs	
70 **kV**	"blue" system 200	"green" system 400
Average	12.5	6.3
Range	8–16	4–8

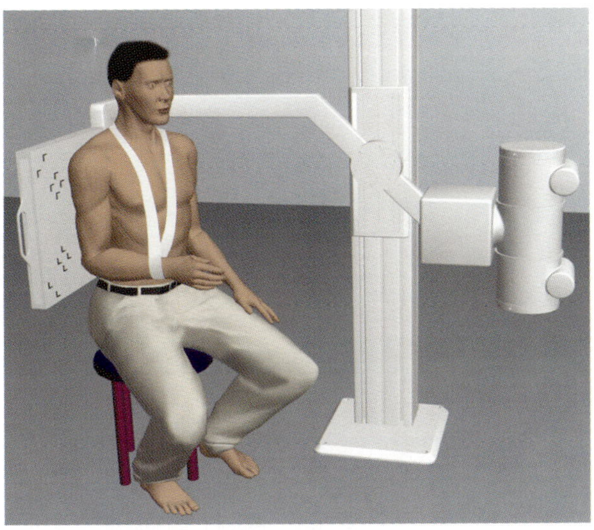

1. Bring in the patient, put the cassette in the cassette holder. Collimate to the format.
2. Position the patient. The patients forearm should be at right angles to the cassette holder, pointing straight towards the x-ray tube.
3. Center and collimate further, if possible.
4. Expose.

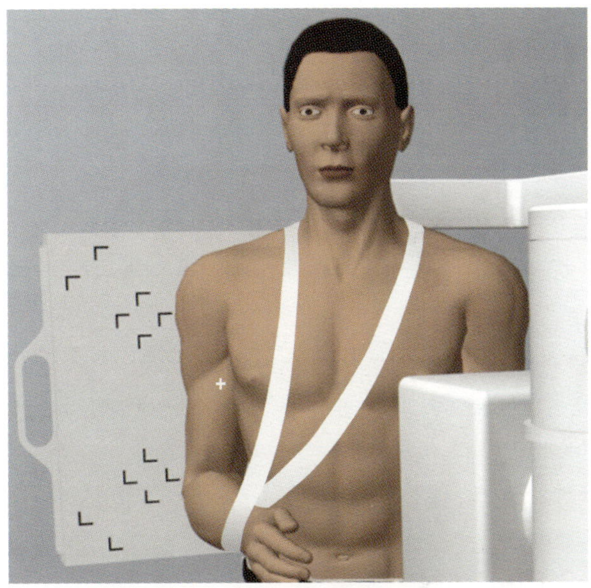

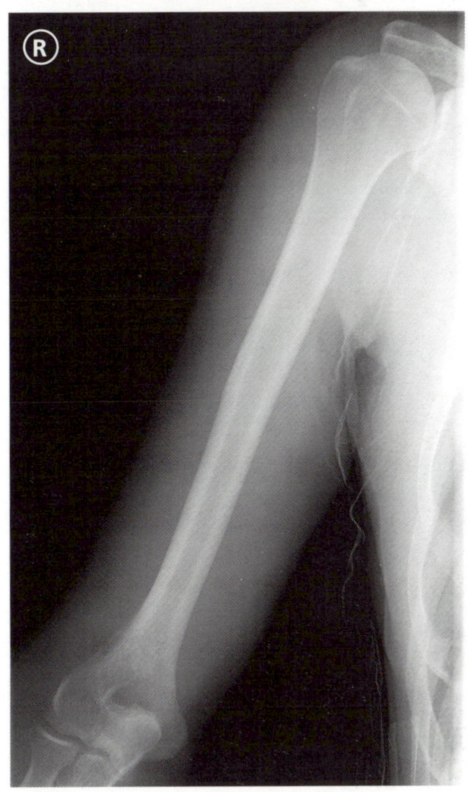

HUMERUS LATERAL – after injury **Sitting erect** ADDITIONAL

Cassette speed
Cassette with screen-film combination, nominal speed 200/400 in the cassette holder

Cassette size
18×43 cm (7×17 inches) or 20×40 cm
Use a **R**ight or **L**eft marker

Exposure values	mAs	
70 **kV**	"blue" system 200	"green" system 400
Average	25	12.5
Range	20–40	10–20

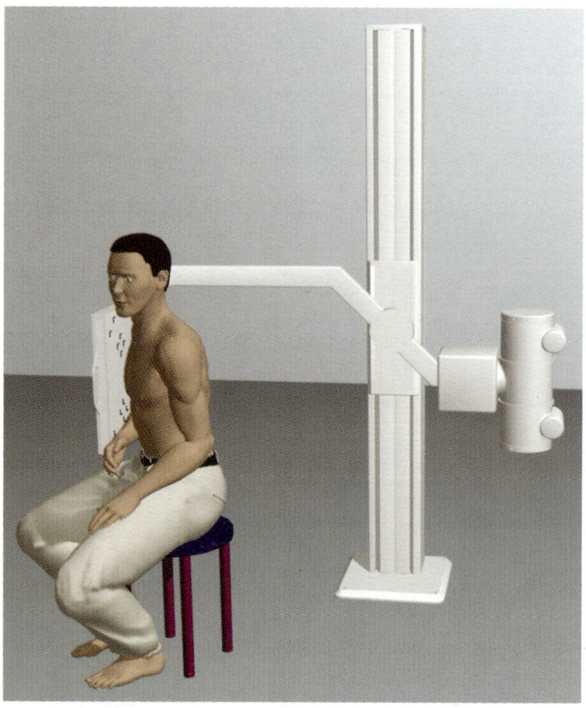

1. Bring in the patient, put the cassette in the cassette holder. Collimate to the format.
2. Position the patient. The patients forearm should be close to the cassette holder.
3. Center and collimate further, if possible.
4. Expose.

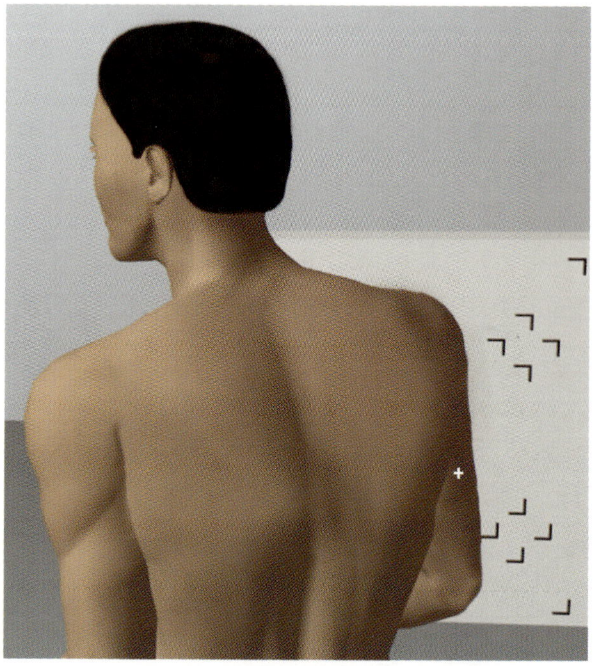

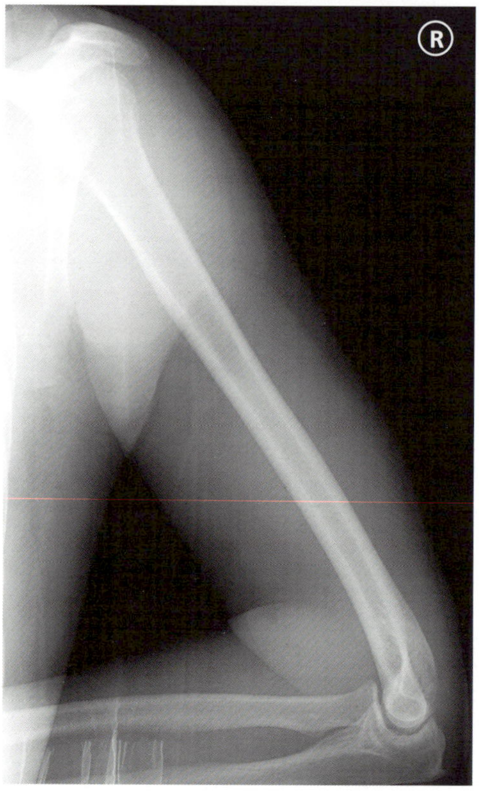

ELBOW AP Sitting, with the arm in supination BASIC

Cassette speed
Cassette with screen-film combination, nominal speed 50/100 on the cassette holder

Cassette size
18×24 cm (8×10 inches)
Half the cassette may be covered by a lead sheet as shown in ARM 22.
Use a **R**ight or **L**eft marker

Exposure values	mAs	
53 kV	"blue" system 50	"green" system 100/63
Average	12.5	10
Range	8–25	6.3–20

1. Bring in the patient, put the cassette on the cassette holder. Collimate to the format.
2. Position the patient. The palm of the patients hand should be facing up. When x-raying a CHILD, if the arm is not long enough for the elbow to reach the centre point of the cassette holder put the cassette on top of a firm support (10–12 cm high) on the cassette holder.
3. Center and collimate further, if possible.
4. Expose.

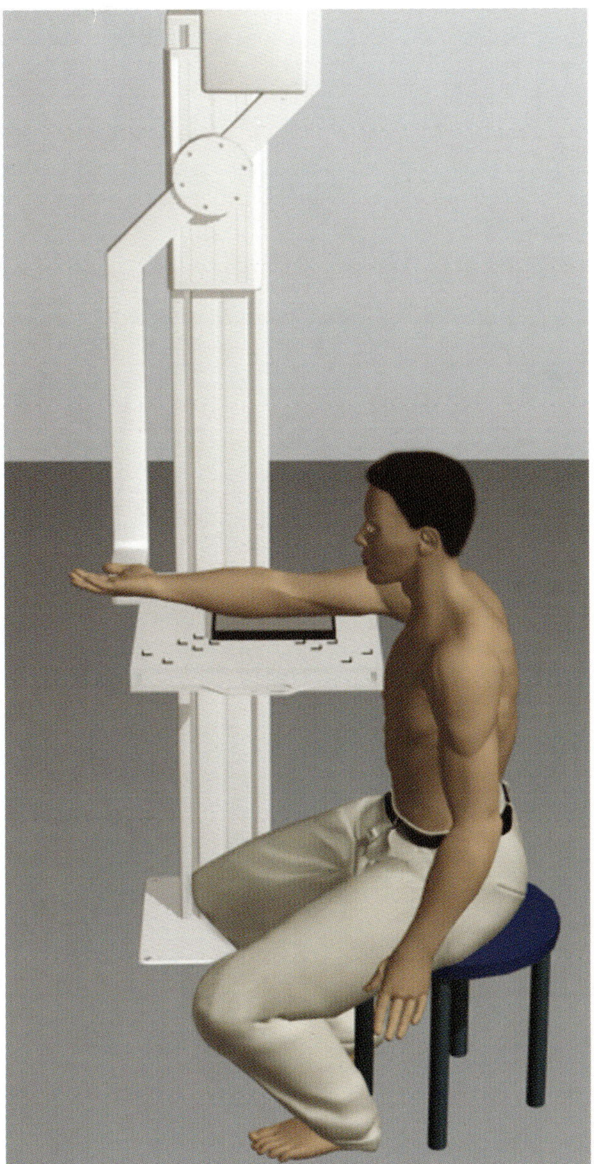

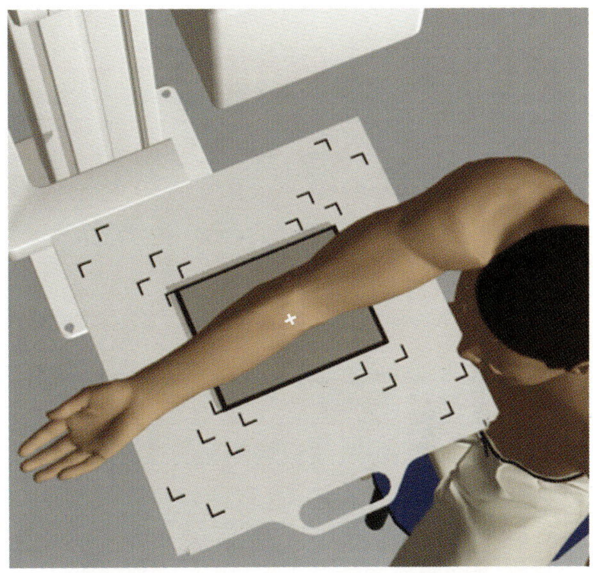

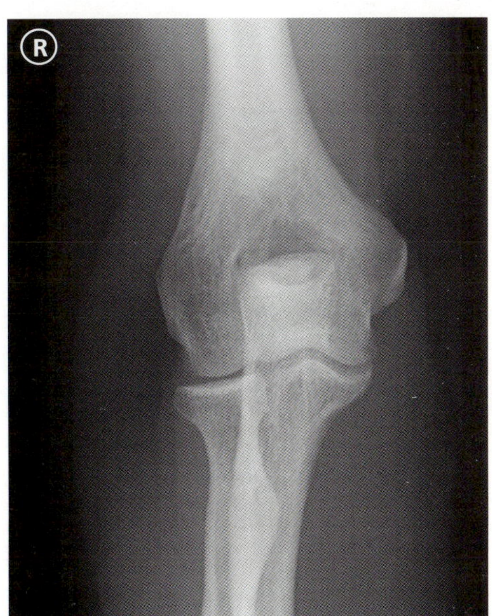

ELBOW LATERAL Sitting, with the arm in supination BASIC

Cassette speed
Cassette with screen-film combination, nominal speed 50/100 on the cassette holder

Cassette size
18×24 cm (8×10 inches)
Half the cassette may be covered by a lead sheet as shown in ARM 22.
Use a **R**ight or **L**eft marker

Exposure values	mAs	
53 **kV**	"blue" system 50	"green" system 100/63
Average	20	16
Range	12.5–25	10–20

1. Bring in the patient, put the cassette on the cassette holder. Collimate to the format.
2. Position the patient. The thumb should be facing up. When x-raying a CHILD, if the arm is not long enough for the elbow to reach the centre point of the cassette holder put the cassette on top of a firm support (10–12 cm high) on the cassette holder.
3. Center and collimate further, if possible.
4. Expose.

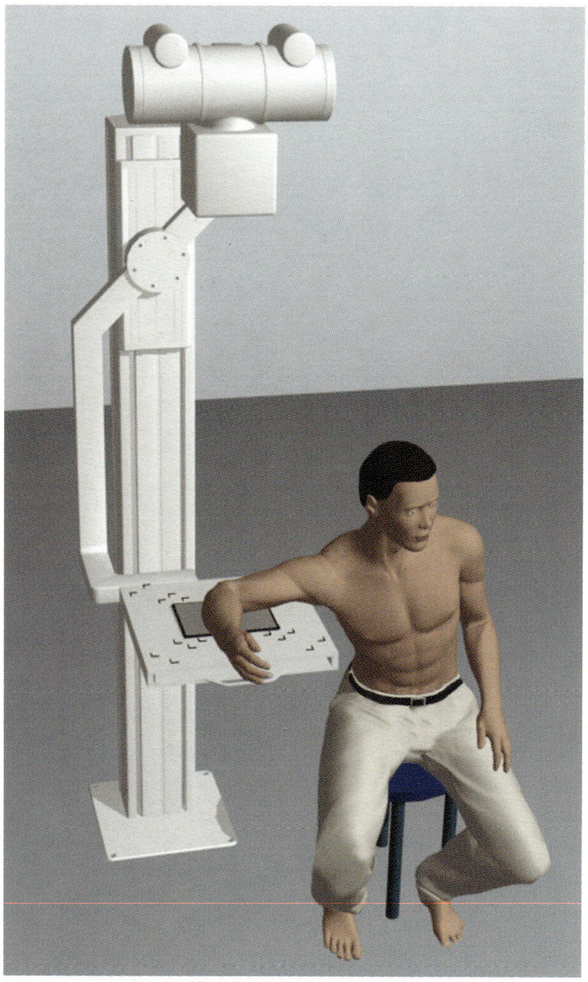

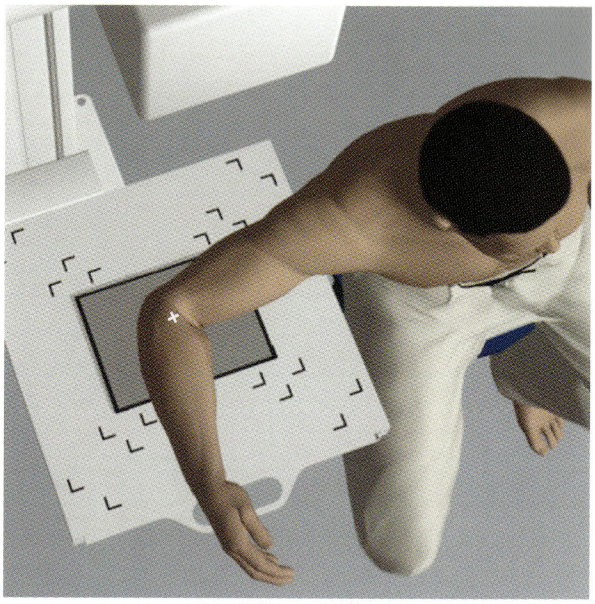

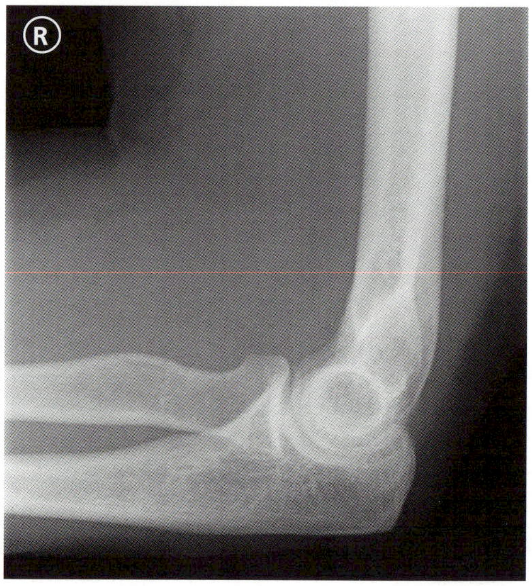

ELBOW AP – after injury **Semiflexed** ADDITIONAL

Sitting, with the arm in supination – two views

Cassette speed
Cassette with screen-film combination, nominal speed 50/100 on the cassette holder

Cassette size
18×24 cm (8×10 inches)
Half the cassette may be covered by a lead sheet as shown in ARM 22.
Use a **R**ight or **L**eft marker

Exposure values	mAs	
53 kV	"blue" system 50	"green" system 100/63
Average	20	16
Range	12.5–25	10–20

1. Bring in the patient, put the cassette on the cassette holder. Collimate to the format.
2. Position the patient. The palm of the patients hand should (if possible) be facing up. When x-raying a CHILD, if the arm is not long enough for the elbow to reach the centre point of the cassette holder put the cassette on top of a firm support (10–12 cm high) on the cassette holder.
3. Center and collimate further, if possible.
4. Expose.
5. Change cassette and take the other view.

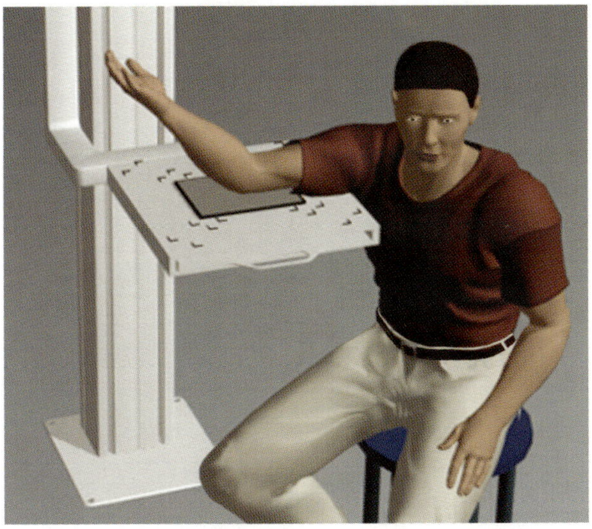

Upper arm parallel to the cassette holder

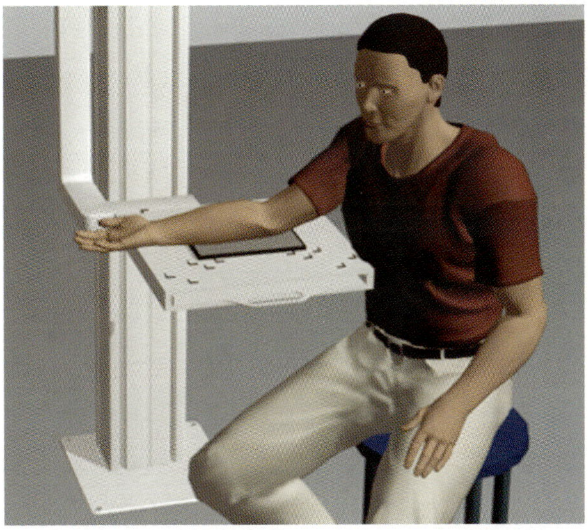

Lower arm parallel to the cassette holder

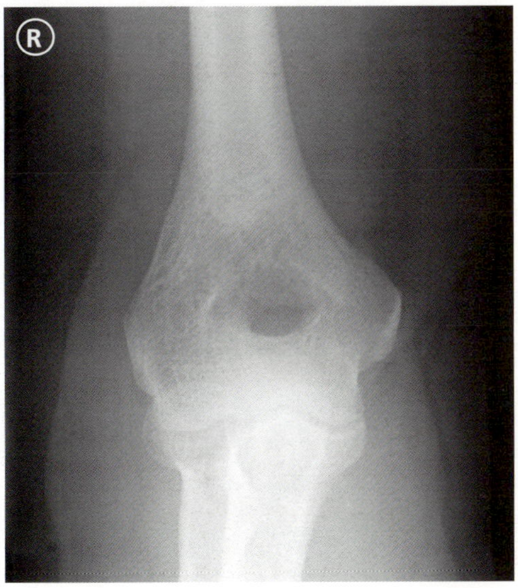

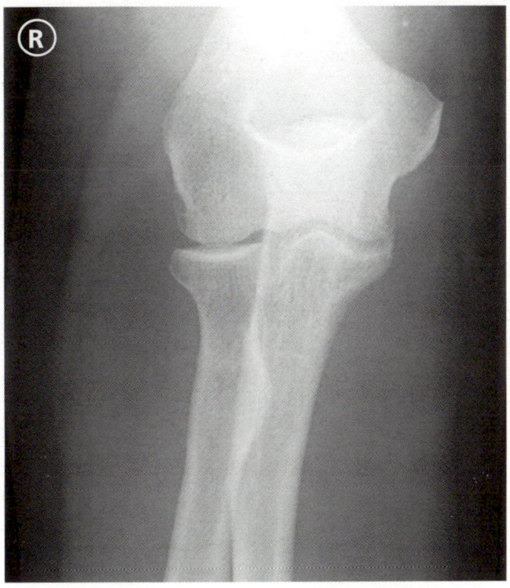

FOREARM PA – after injury   Sitting – with the arm in supination   BASIC

Cassette speed
Cassette with screen-film combination, nominal speed 50/100 on the cassette holder. If the arm is in plaster, nominal speed 200/400.

Cassette size
24×30 (10×12 inches)
18×24 cm (8×10 inches) for a child
Use a **R**ight or **L**eft marker

Exposure values	mAs	
53 **kV**	"blue" system 50	"green" system 100/63
Average	12.5	10
Range	8–20	6.3–16
In plaster 60 **kV**	"blue" system 200	"green" system 400/320
Average	6.3	4

1. Bring in the patient, put the cassette on the cassette holder. Collimate to the format.
2. Position the patient. The palm of the patients hand should be facing down, the elbow bent at right angle as shown and the upper arm parallel to the cassette holder.
3. Center and collimate further, if possible.
4. Expose.

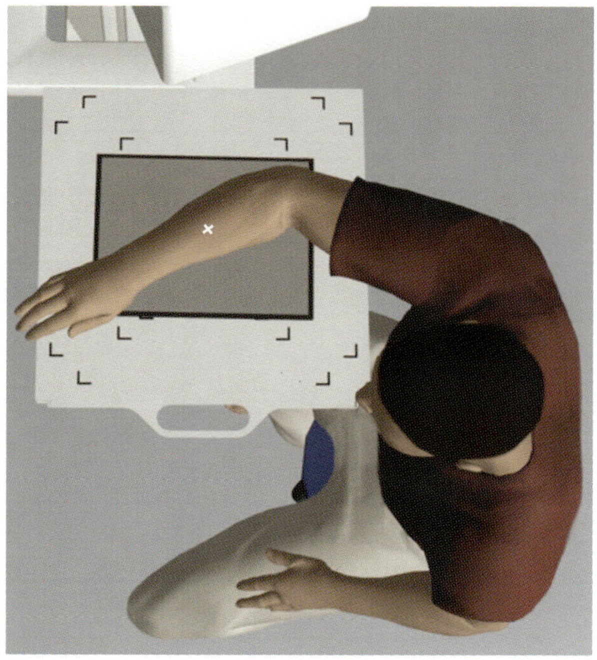

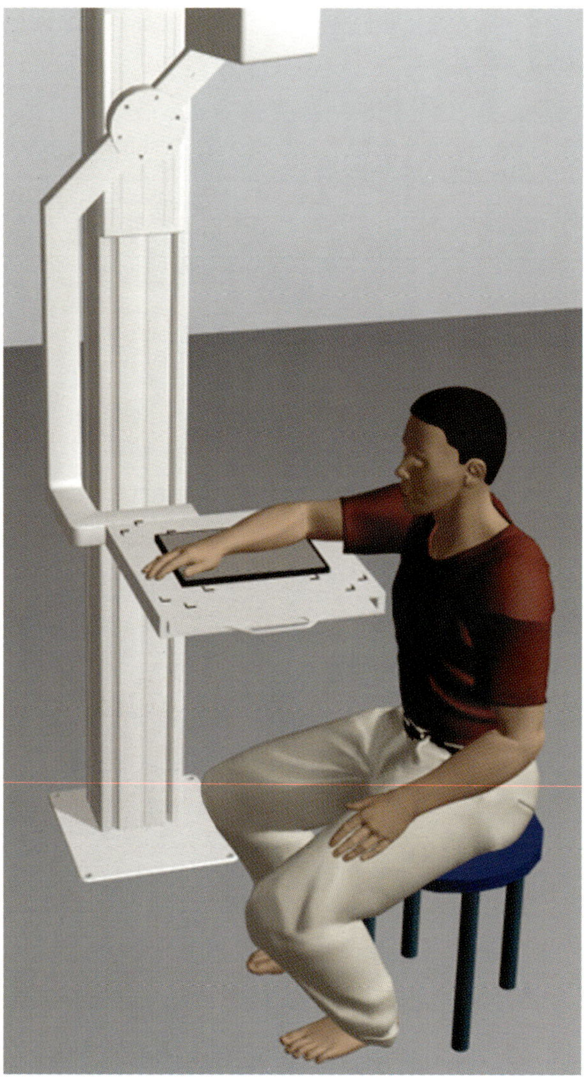

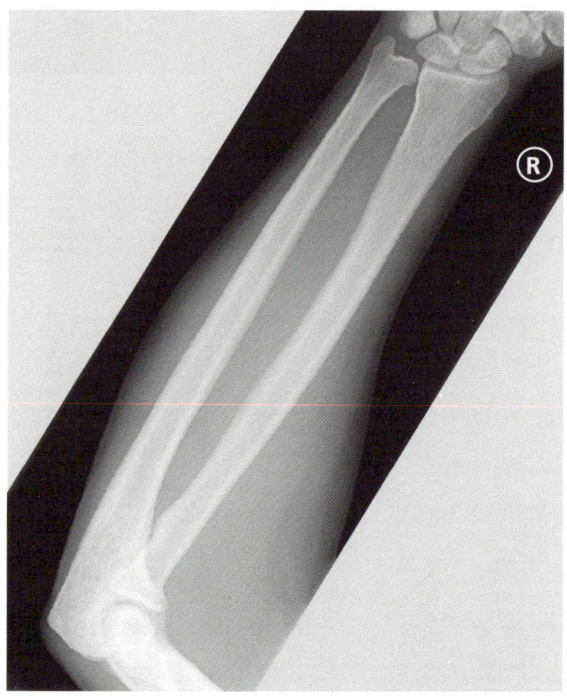

FOREARM LATERAL – after injury   Standing or sitting   BASIC

Cassette speed
Cassette with screen-film combination, nominal speed 50/100 on the cassette holder. If the arm is in plaster, nominal speed 200/400.

Cassette size
24×30 (10×12 inches)
18×24 cm (8×10 inches) for a child
Use a **R**ight or **L**eft marker

Exposure values	mAs	
53 **kV**	"blue" system 50	"green" system 100/63
Average	12.5	10
Range	8–20	6.3–16
In plaster 60 **kV**	"blue" system 200	"green" system 400/320
Average	6.3	4

1. Bring in the patient, put the cassette on the cassette holder. Collimate to the format.
2. Position the patient. Standing or sitting (whichever is more comfortable for the patient). The thumb should be uppermost.
3. Center and collimate further, if possible.
4. Expose.

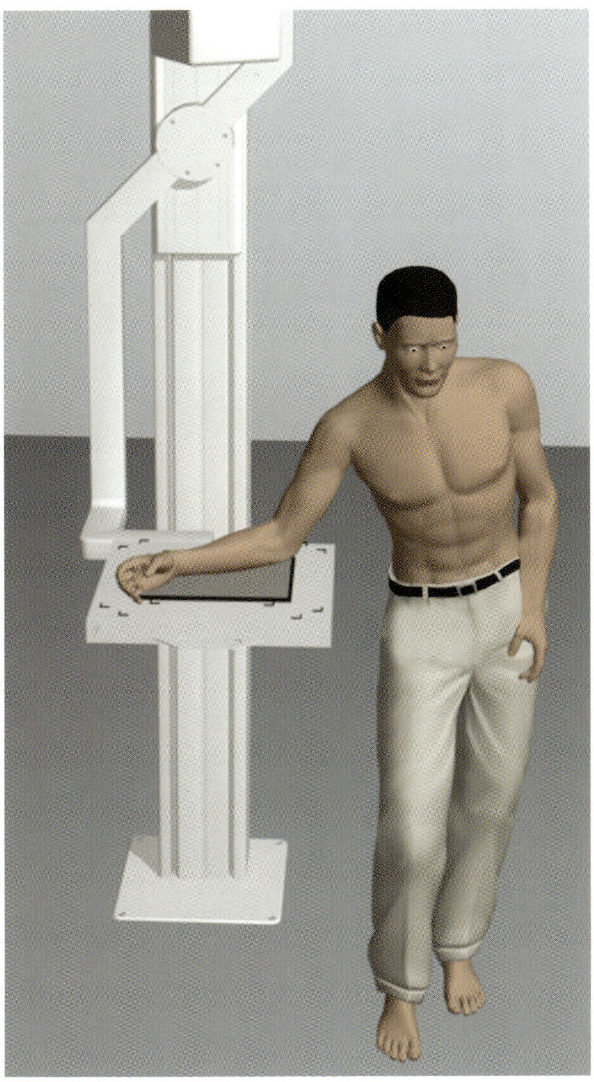

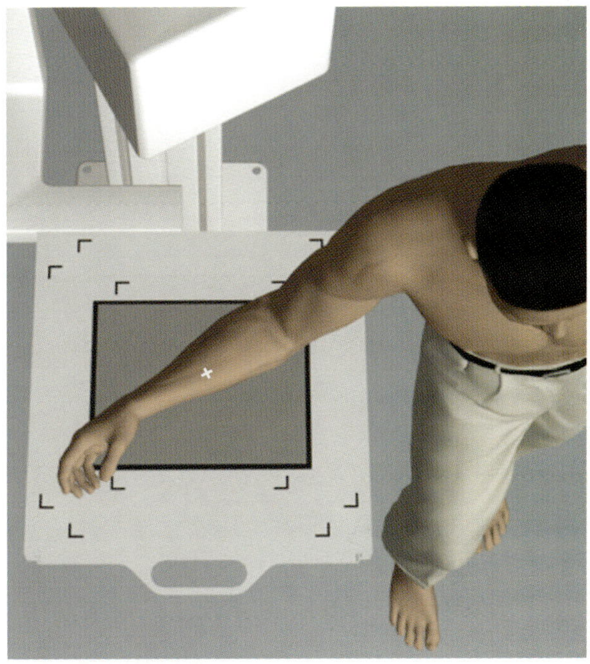

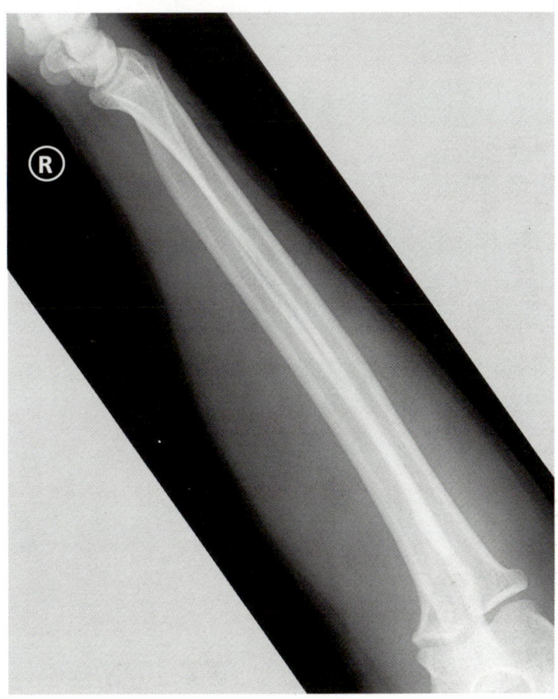

WRIST PA Sitting – with hand turned as shown BASIC
Ulnar deviation ADDITIONAL

Cassette speed
Cassette with screen-film combination, nominal speed 50/100 on the cassette holder

Cassette size
18×24 cm (8×10 inches)
Half the cassette may be covered by a lead sheet as shown in ARM 22.
Use a **R**ight or **L**eft marker

Exposure values	mAs	
53 **kV**	"blue" system 50	"green" system 100/63
Average	8	6.3
Range	5–16	4–12.5

1. Bring in the patient, put the cassette on the cassette holder. Collimate to the format.
2. Position the patient. The palm of the patients hand facing down.
3. Center and collimate further, if possible.
4. Expose.
5. On the request of the doctor, change cassette and position as shown for ulnar deviation and make a new exposure.

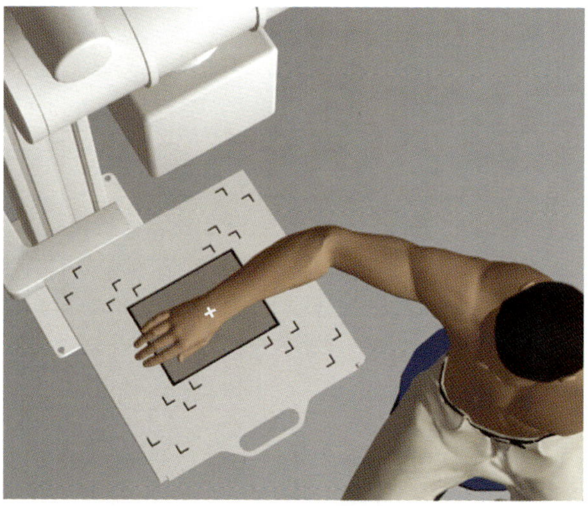

BASIC

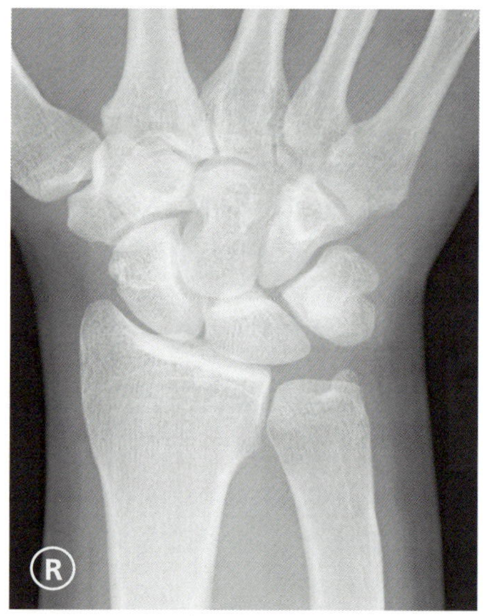

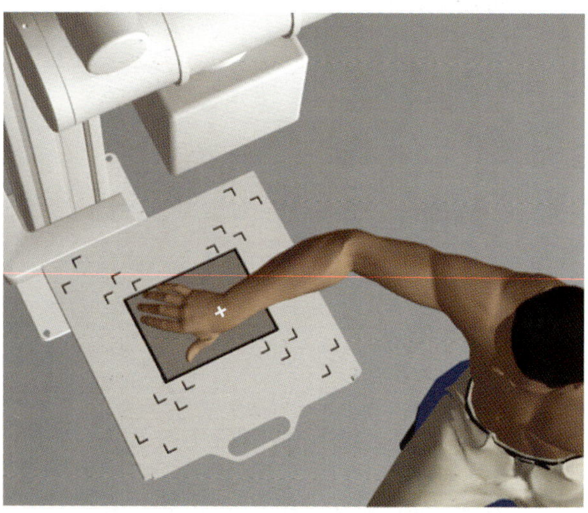

Ulnar deviation ADDITIONAL

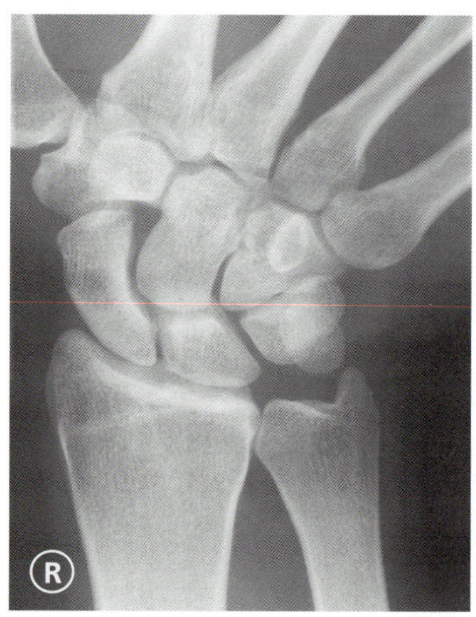

WRIST LATERAL Standing or sitting BASIC

Cassette speed
Cassette with screen-film combination, nominal speed 50/100 on the cassette holder.

Cassette size
18×24 cm (8×10 inches)
Half the cassette may be covered by a lead sheet as shown in ARM 22.
Use a **R**ight or **L**eft marker

Exposure values	mAs	
53 **kV**	"blue" system 50	"green" system 100/63
Average	12.5	10
Range	8–20	6.3–16

1. Bring in the patient, put the cassette on the cassette holder. Collimate to the format.
2. Position the patient. Standing or sitting (whichever is more comfortable for the patient). The thumb uppermost.
3. Center and collimate further, if possible.
4. Expose.

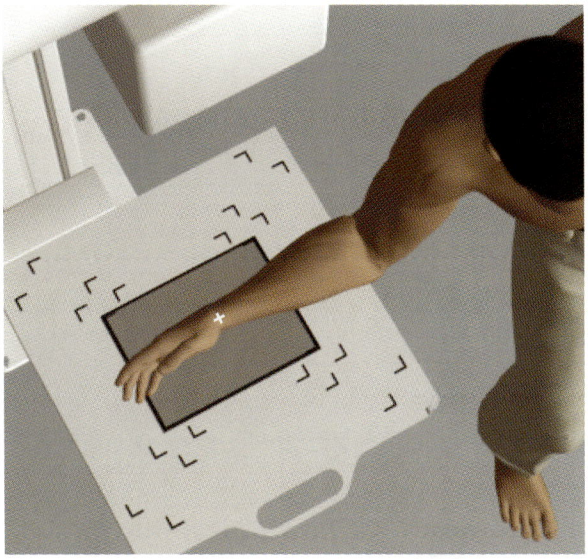

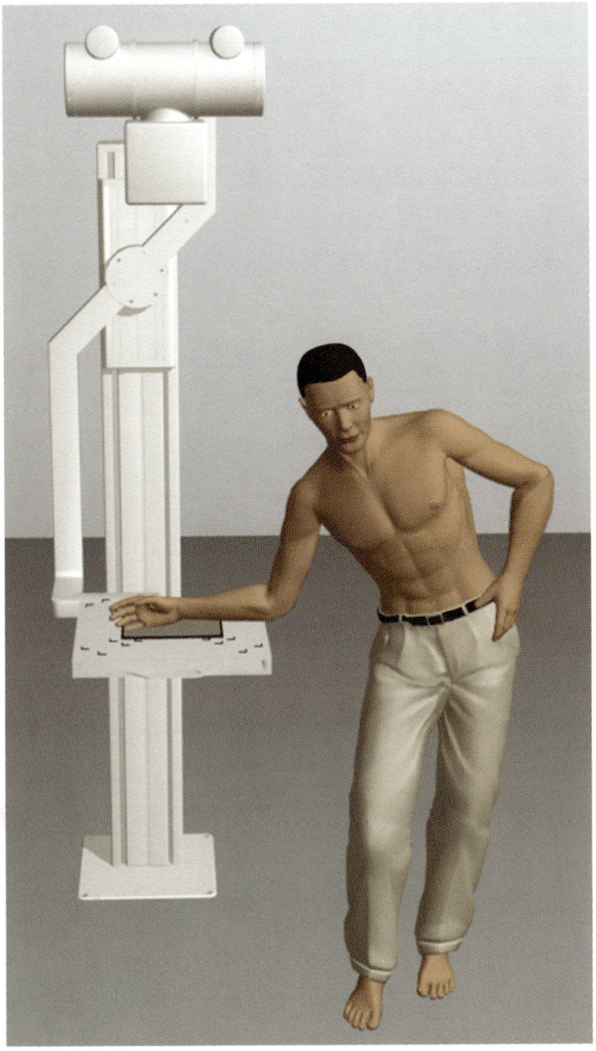

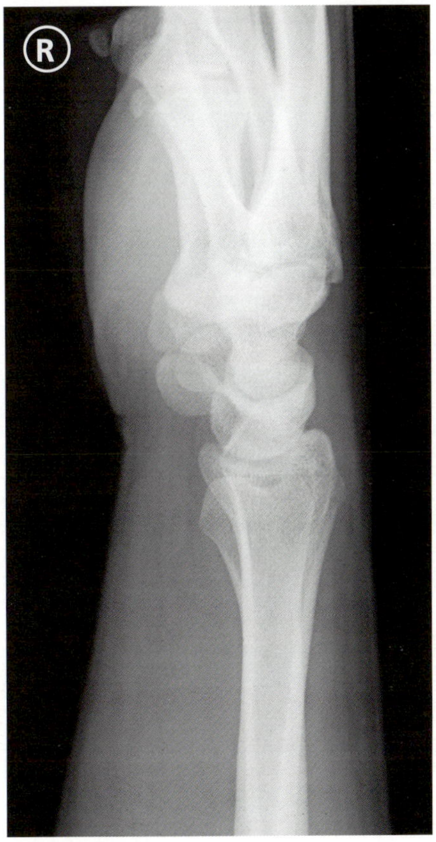

SCAPHOID – after injury **Sitting** ADDITIONAL

Two views

Cassette speed
Cassette with screen-film combination, nominal speed 50/100 on the cassette holder

Cassette size
18×24 cm (8×10 inches)
Half the cassette may be covered by a lead sheet as shown in ARM 22.
Use a **R**ight or **L**eft marker

Exposure values	mAs	
53 **kV**	"blue" system 50	"green" system 100/63
Average	10	8
Range	6.3–20	5–16

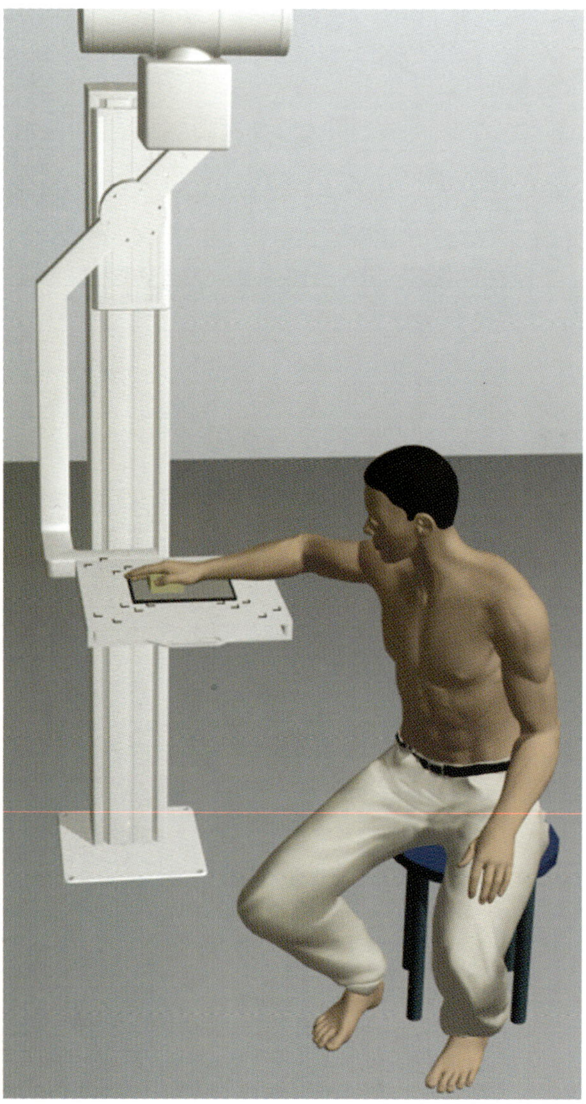

1. Bring in the patient, put the cassette on the cassette holder. Collimate to the format.
2. Position the patient. The palm of the hand with ulnar deviation, resting on a supporting pad, as shown.
3. Center and collimate further, if possible.
4. Expose.
5. Take the other view.

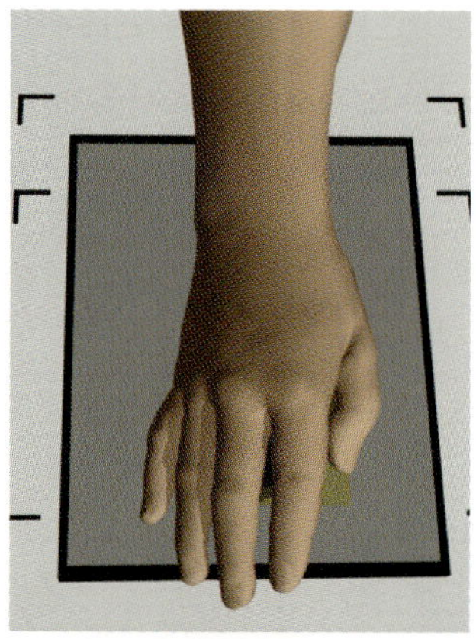

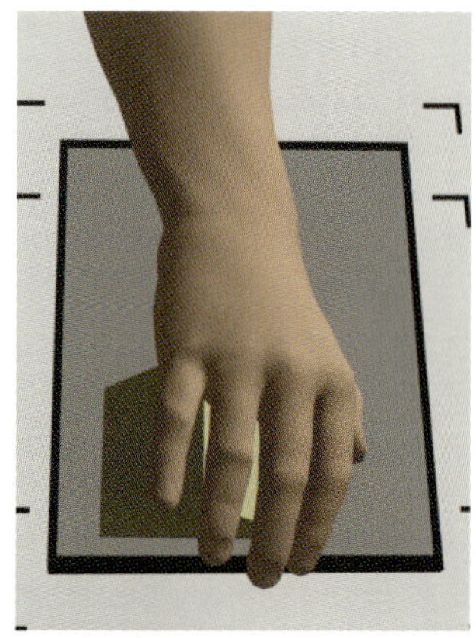

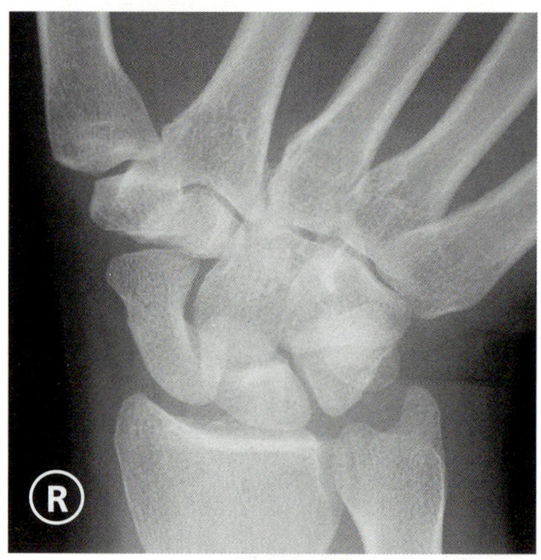

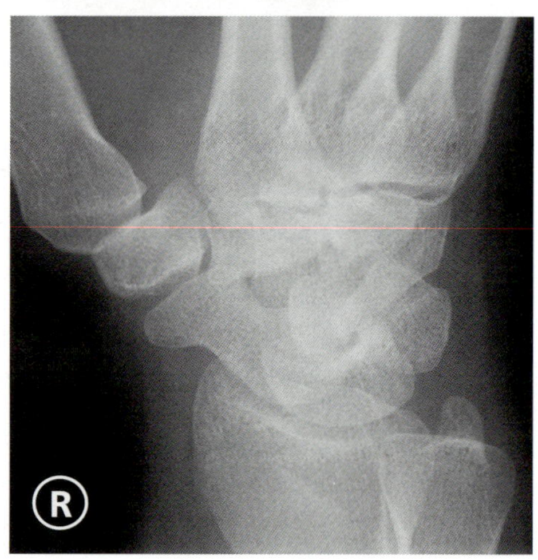

HAND PA and OBLIQUES Sitting BASIC (PA) ADDITIONAL (obliques)

Cassette speed
Cassette with screen-film combination, nominal speed 50/100 on the cassette holder

Cassette size
18×24 cm (8×10 inches)
Half the cassette may be covered by a lead sheet as shown in ARM 22.
Use a **R**ight or **L**eft marker

Exposure values	mAs	
46 **kV**	"blue" system 50	"green" system 100/50
Average	8	8
Range	5–12.5	5–12.5

1. Bring in the patient, put the cassette on the cassette holder. Collimate to the format.
2. Position the patient. The palm of the patients hand facing down. Center and collimate further, if possible.
3. Expose.
4. On the request of the doctor, change cassette and position as shown for PA and AP obliques and make new exposures.

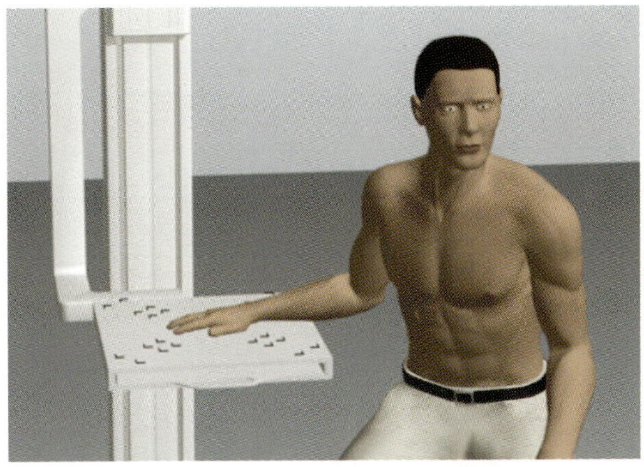

Basic PA

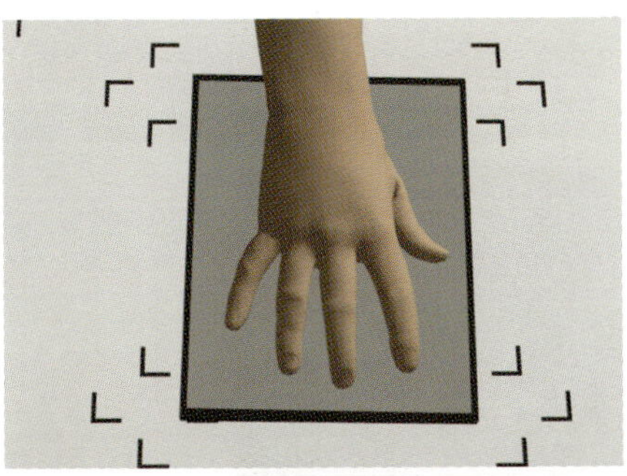

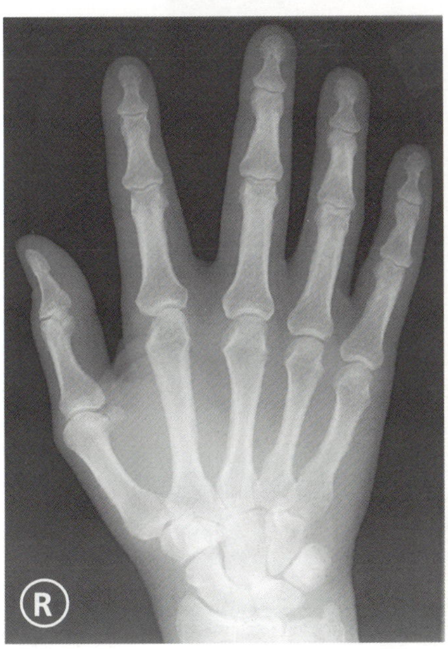

Obliques

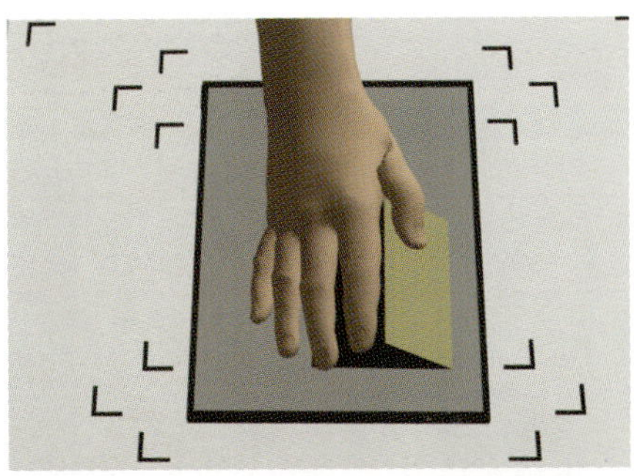

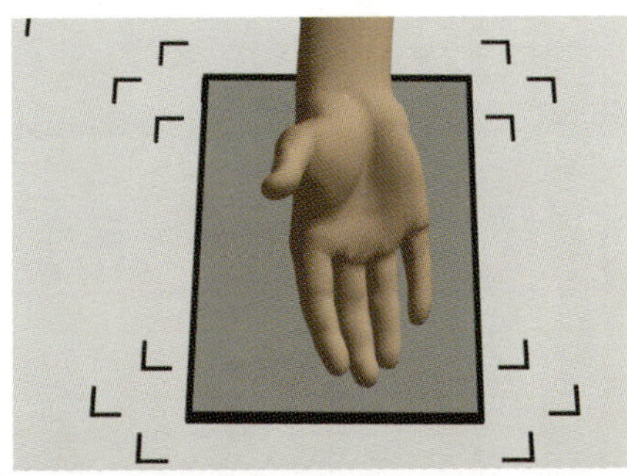

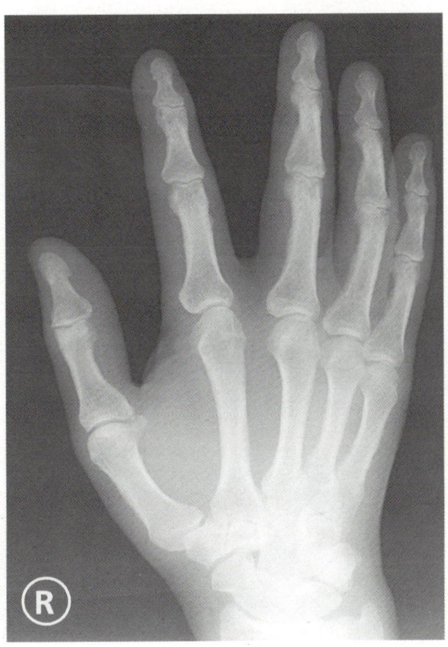

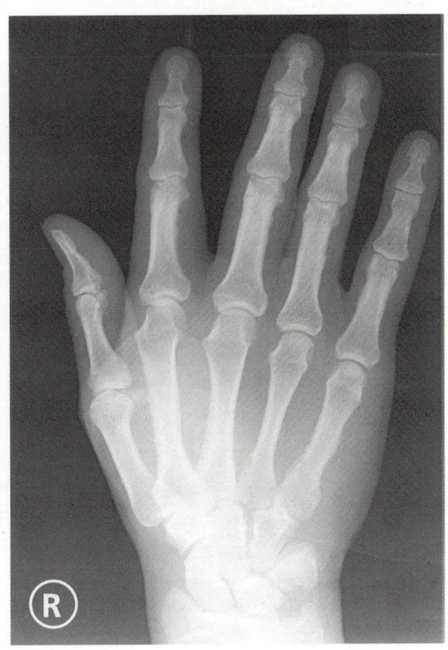

THUMB AP Standing BASIC

Cassette speed
Cassette with screen-film combination, nominal speed 50/100 on the cassette holder

Cassette size
18×24 cm (8×10 inches)
Half the cassette can be used for AP, the other for lateral thumb. Protect the other part of the cassette with a lead strip as shown in ARM 22.
Use a **R**ight or **L**eft marker

1. Bring in the patient, put the cassette on the cassette holder. Collimate to the format.
2. Position the patient. The thumb on the cassette.
3. Center and collimate further, if possible.
4. Expose.

Exposure values	mAs	
46 **kV**	"blue" system 50	"green" system 100/50
Average	16	16
Range	12.5–25	12.5–25

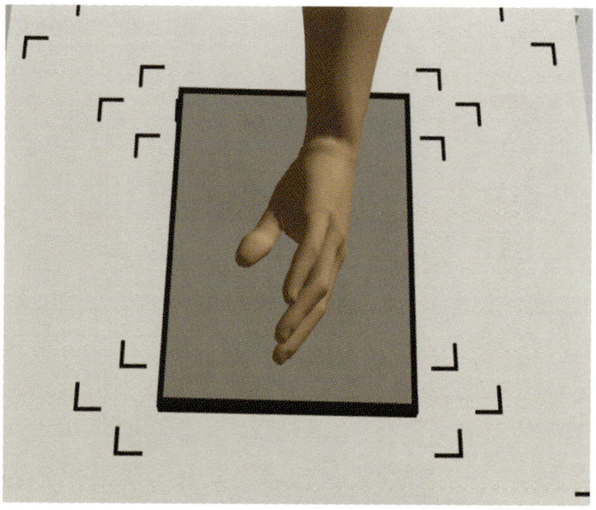

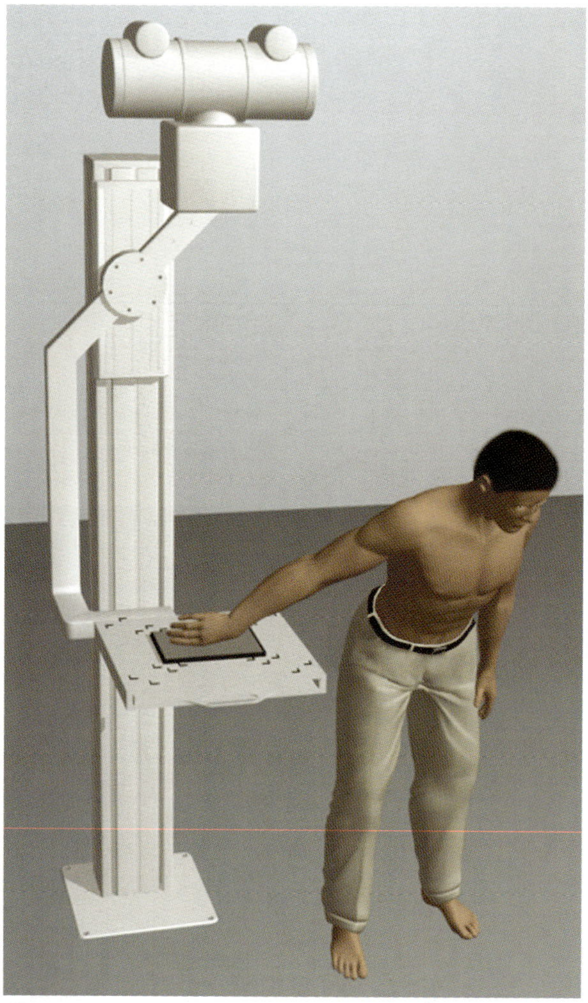

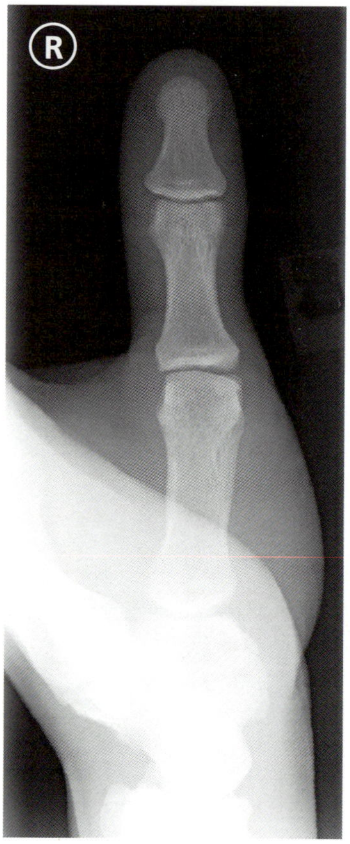

THUMB LATERAL Sitting or standing BASIC

Cassette speed
Cassette with screen-film combination, nominal speed 50/100 on the cassette holder

Cassette size
18×24 cm (8×10 inches)
Half the cassette can be used for AP the other for lateral thumb. Protect the other part of the cassette with a lead strip.
Use a **R**ight or **L**eft marker

Exposure values	mAs	
46 **kV**	"blue" system 50	"green" system 100/50
Average	16	16
Range	12.5–25	12.5–25

1. Bring in the patient, put the cassette on the cassette holder. Collimate to the format.
2. Position the patient. The palm of the patients hand facing down, fingers closed.
3. Center and collimate further, if possible.
4. Expose.

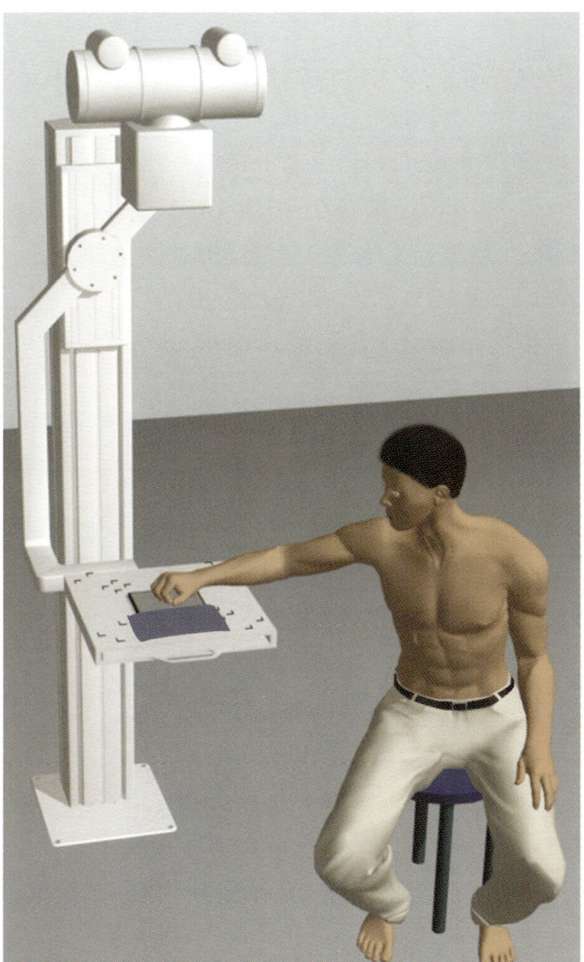

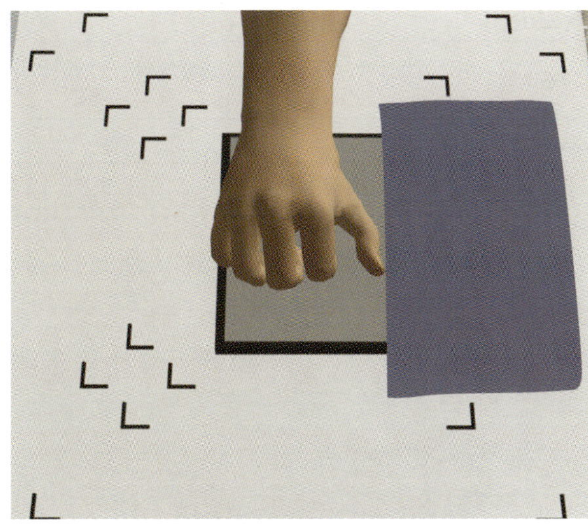

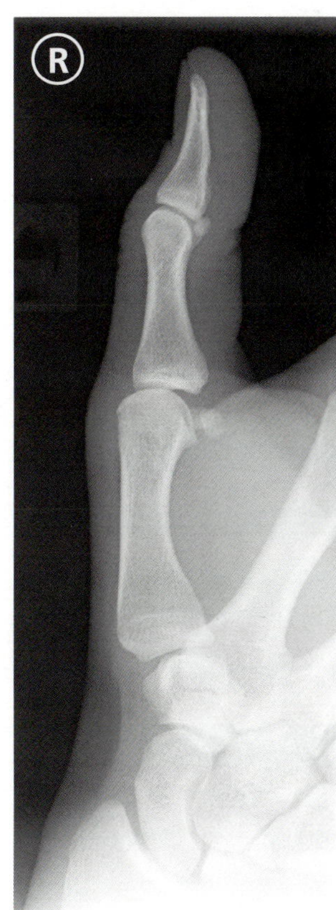

SINGLE FINGER LATERAL Sitting or standing BASIC

Cassette speed
Cassette with screen-film combination, nominal speed 50/100 on the cassette holder

Cassette size
18×24 cm (8×10 inches)
Half the cassette can be used for each finger. Protect the other part of the cassette with a lead strip.
Use a **R**ight or **L**eft marker

Exposure values	mAs	
46 **kV**	"blue" system 50	"green" system 100/50
Average	8	8
Range	6.3–12.5	6.3–12.5

1. Bring in the patient, put the cassette on the cassette holder, cover half the cassette with a lead sheet. Collimate to the format.
2. Position the patient. If possible extend the finger to be examined with a stick as shown. Center and collimate further, if possible.
3. Expose.
4. Hand (ARM 21) is used for AP and obliques.
5. The radiograph below shows separate view of the third finger.

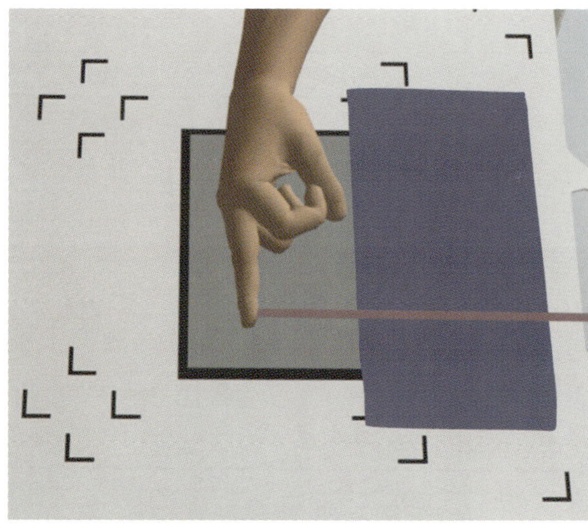

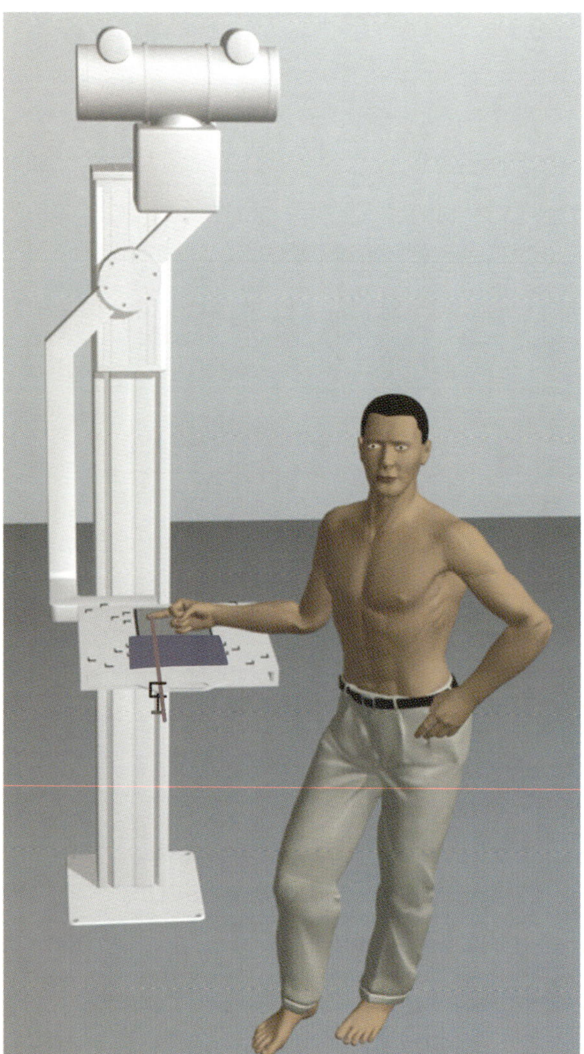

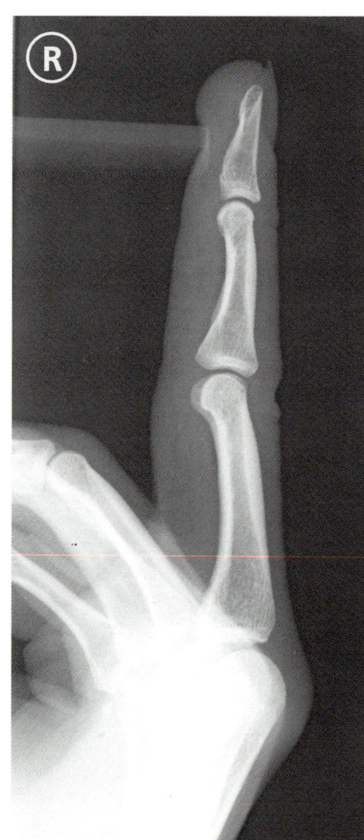

Leg

With some exceptions X-rays of the leg are taken with the patient lying supine.

PELVIS AP **Supine** BASIC

Cassette speed
Cassette with screen-film combination, nominal speed 200/400 in the cassette holder

Cassette size
35×43 (14×17 inches)
Use a **R**ight or **L**eft marker

Exposure values	mAs	
70 **kV**	"blue" system 200	"green" system 400
Average	100	50
Range	40–200	20–100

1. Bring in the patient, put the cassette in the cassette holder. Collimate to that format.
2. Position the patient. If the patient is INJURED, do not move the feet.
   If the patient is NOT INJURED, turn the feet with heels apart and toes together as shown.
3. Center 4 cm above the symphysis and collimate further, if possible.
4. Expose.

For INFANTS and SMALL CHILDREN use LEG 25

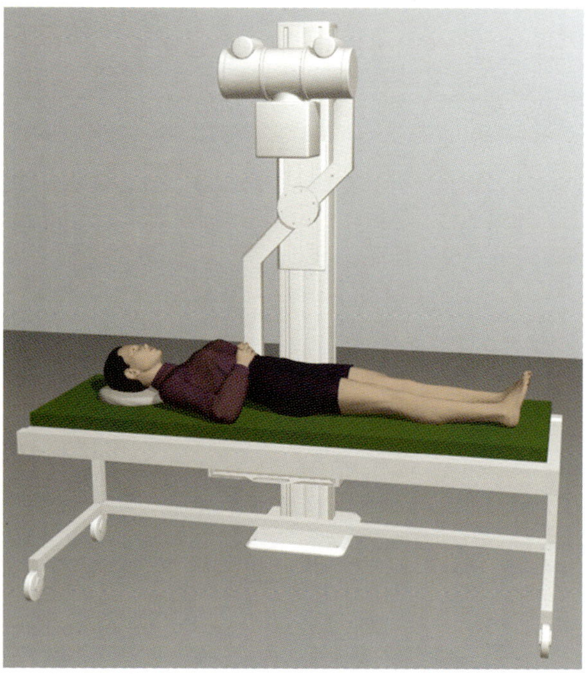

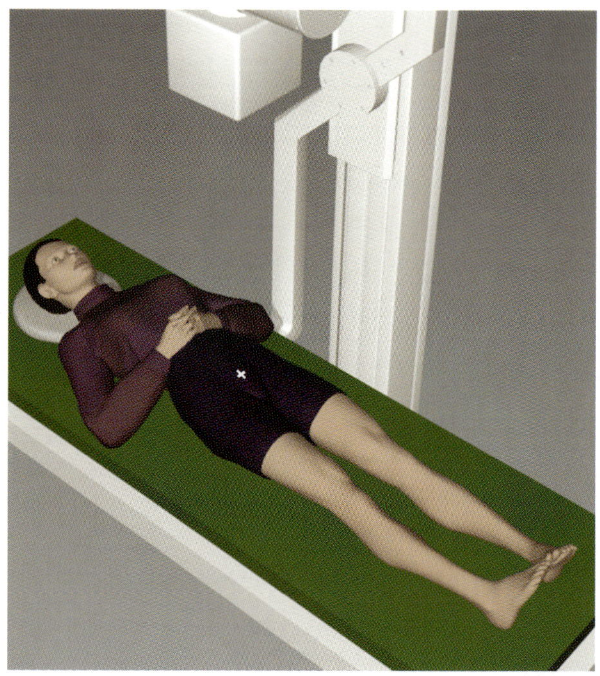

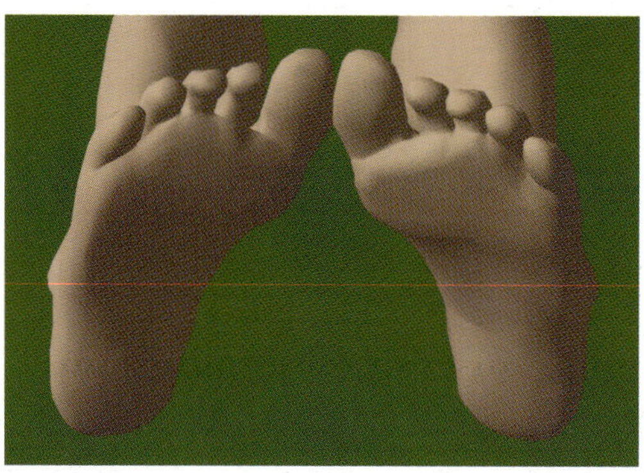

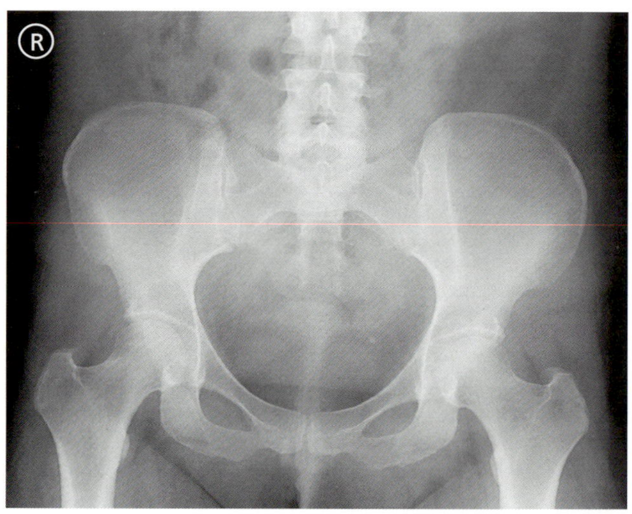

HIP JOINT AP Supine BASIC

Cassette speed
Cassette with screen-film combination, nominal speed 200/400 in the cassette holder

Cassette size
24×30 cm (10×12 inches)
18×24 cm (8×10 inches) for a child
Use a **R**ight or **L**eft marker

Exposure values	mAs	
70 **kV**	"blue" system 200	"green" system 400
Average	125	63
Range	63–250	32–125

1. Bring in the patient, put the cassette in the cassette holder. Collimate to that format.
2. Position the patient. If the patient is INJURED, do not move the feet.
   If the patient is NOT INJURED, turn the feet with heels apart and toes together as shown.
3. Center and collimate further, if possible.
4. Expose.

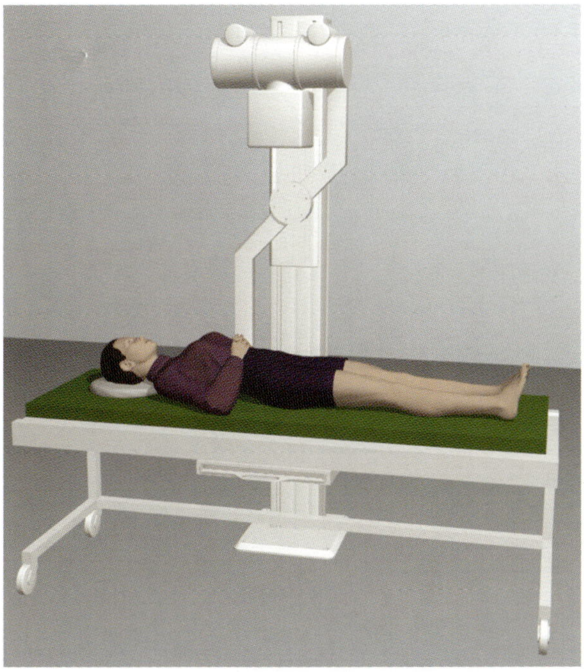

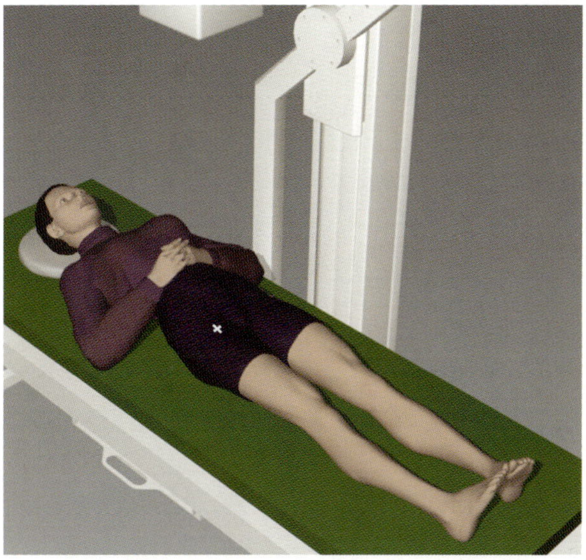

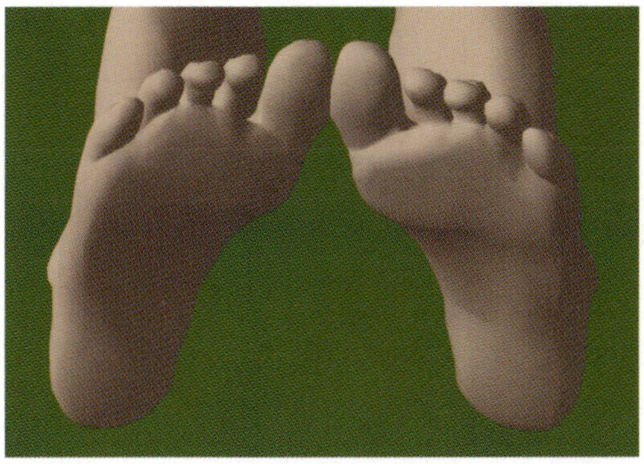

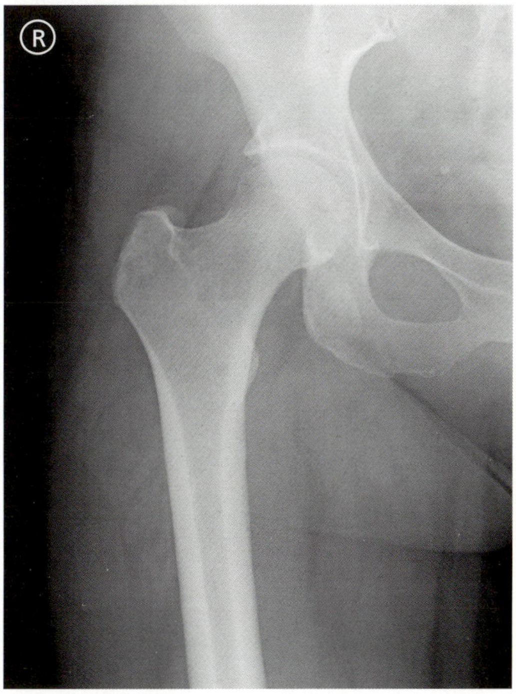

HIP JOINT LATERAL **Supine** BASIC

If a fracture is suspected, see LEG 4 and LEG 5

Cassette speed
Cassette with screen-film combination, nominal speed 200/400 in the cassette holder

Cassette size
24×30 cm (10×12 inches)
Use a **R**ight or **L**eft marker

Exposure values	mAs	
70 **kV**	"blue" system 200	"green" system 400
Average	125	63
Range	63–250	32–125

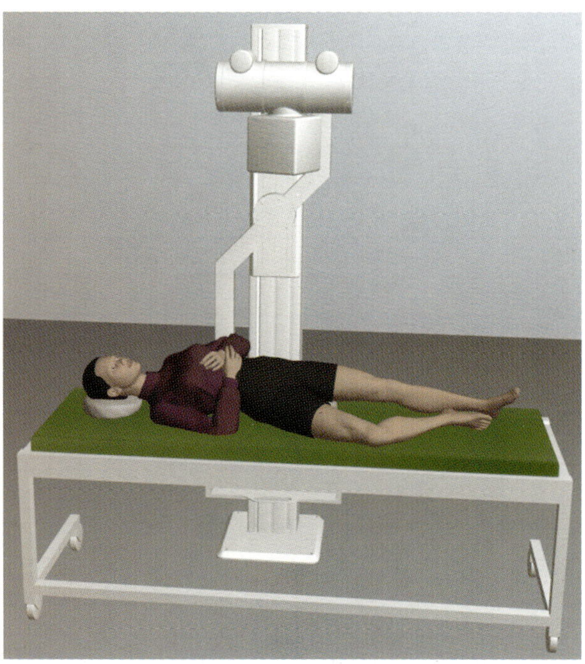

1. Bring in the patient, put the cassette in the cassette holder. Collimate to that format.
2. DO NOT USE IF the patient is INJURED. Position the patient. Turn the leg and the patient carefully on the side to be x-rayed so that the leg is flat on the table.
3. Center and collimate further, if possible.
4. Expose.

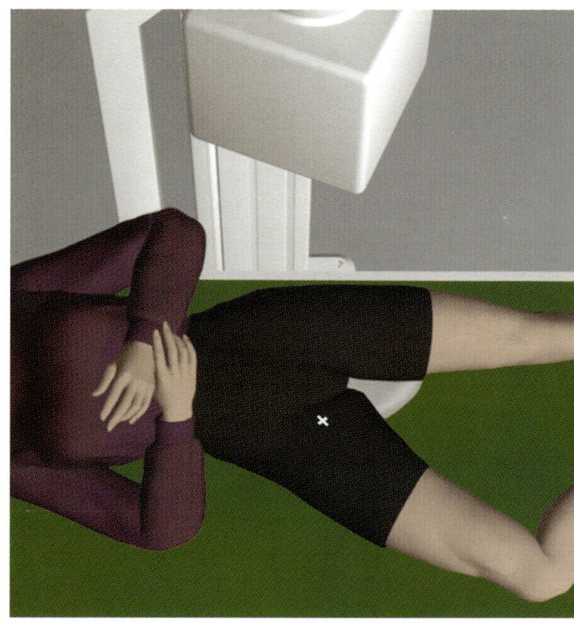

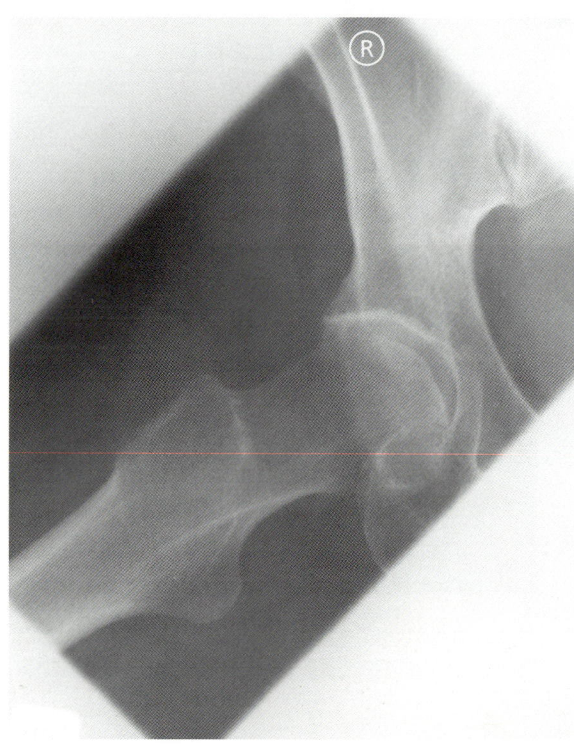

HIP JOINT OBLIQUE LATERAL – if a fracture is suspected Supine ADDITIONAL

Non-conventional lateral view

Cassette speed
Cassette with screen-film combination, nominal speed 200/400 in the cassette holder

Cassette size
24×30 cm (10×12 inches)
Use a **R**ight or **L**eft marker

Exposure values	mAs	
80 kV	"blue" system 200	"green" system 400/450
Average	160	80
Range	100–250	50–160

1. Bring in the patient, put the cassette in the cassette holder. Collimate to that format. This is not the conventional lateral view of the femoral neck.
2. Put the patient and trolley in position, the hip to be examined close to the cassette holder.
3. Angle the tube arm 25° as shown, make sure the lower part of the cassette holder touches the trolley as shown.
4. Center and collimate further, if possible.
5. Expose.

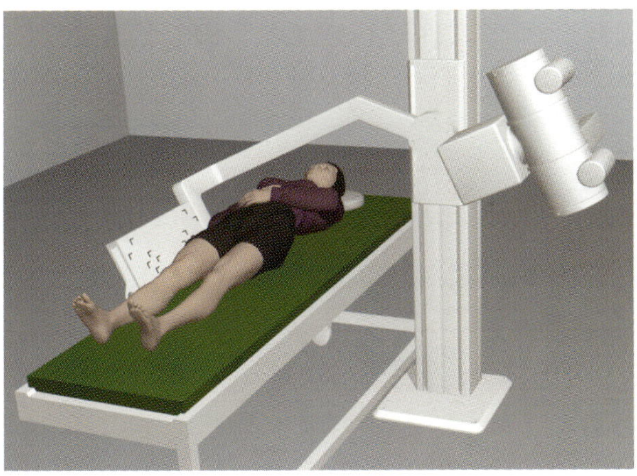

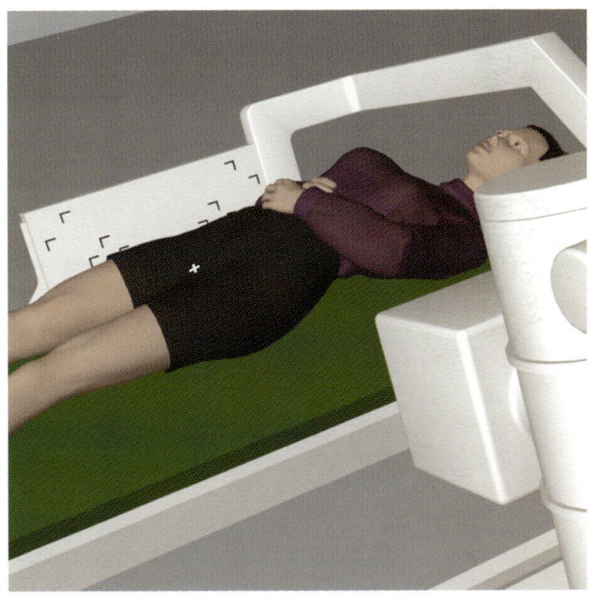

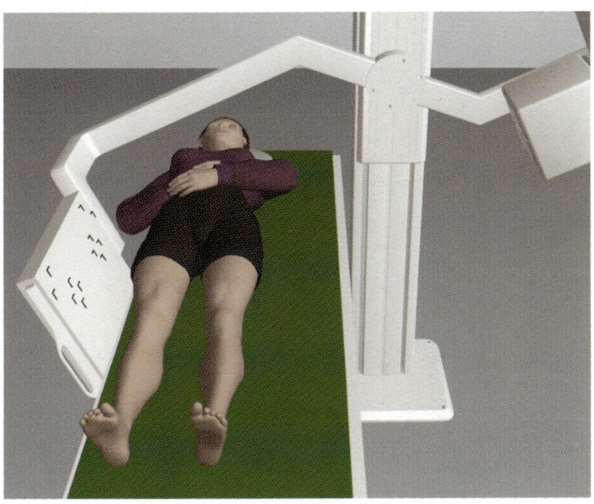

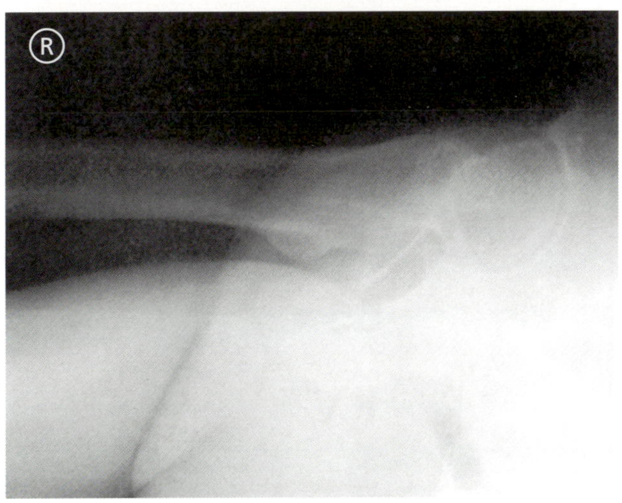

HIP JOINT LATERAL – if a fracture is suspected Supine ADDITIONAL

Conventional lateral view

Cassette speed
Cassette with screen-film combination, nominal speed 200/400 on the table with a loose grid

Cassette size
24×30 cm (10×12 inches)
Use a **R**ight or **L**eft marker

Exposure values	mAs	
kV	"blue" system 90 **kV**; 200	"green" system 80 **kV**; 400/450
Average	160	125
Range	100–250	80–200

1. Bring in the patient. Place the patient on the trolley. Put the cassette close to the hip to be examined, with the patient supporting it.
2. Angle the tube arm 30° and the tube 30° as shown = horizontal beam.
3. Put the patient and trolley in position, angled 30° as shown, the hip to be examined close to the cassette with 120 cm FFD.
4. Let the patient support the cassette with loose grid.
5. Bend the uninjured leg and support it. Center and collimate.
6. Expose.

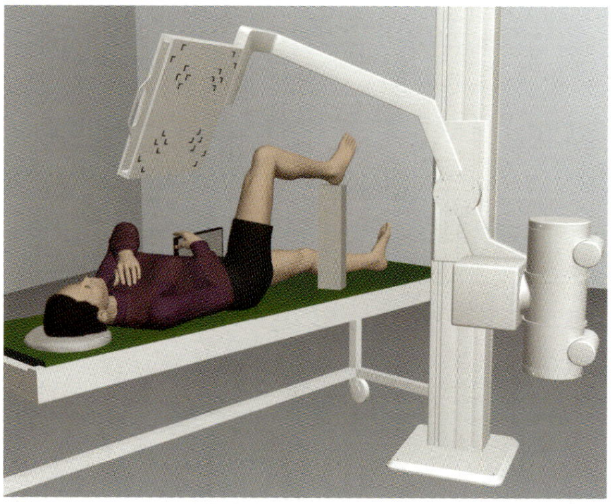

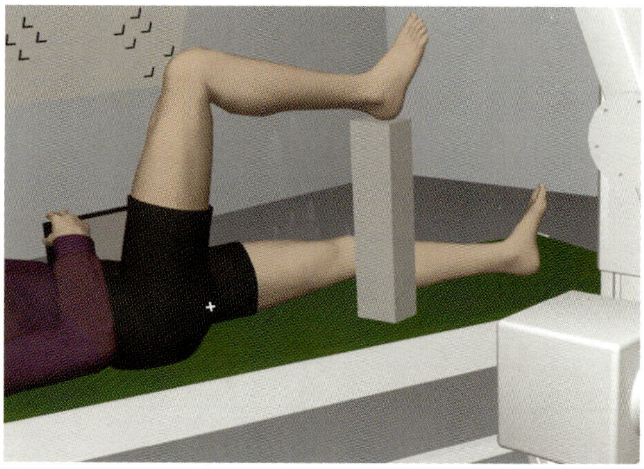

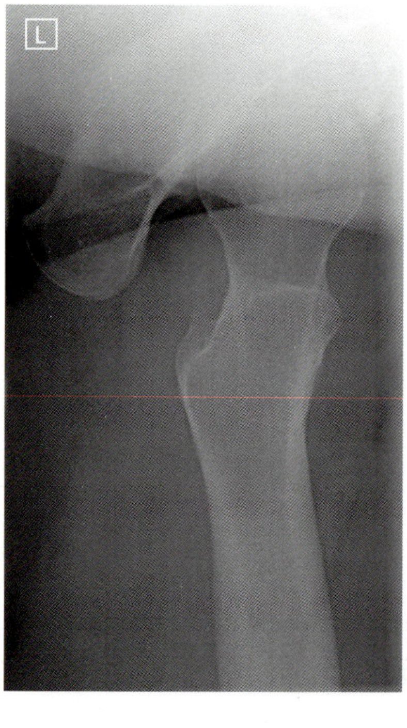

FEMUR AP Supine BASIC

Cassette speed
Cassette with screen-film combination, nominal speed 200/400 in the cassette holder.
For a CHILD, cassette **on** the table

Cassette size
18×43 cm (7×17 inches)
24×30 cm (10×12 inches) for a child
Use a **R**ight or **L**eft marker

Exposure values	mAs	
70 **kV**	"blue" system 200	"green" system 400
Average	50	25
Range	32–100	16–40
Child 53 **kV**	"blue" system 200	"green" system 400/250
Range	3.2–8	2.5–6.3

1. Bring in the patient, put the cassette in the cassette holder (on the table for a child). Collimate to the format.
2. Position the patient. If the patient is INJURED, do not move the feet. The joint nearest to the injury has to be visible.
   If the patient is NOT INJURED, turn the feet with heels apart and toes together as shown. The hip joint and/or the knee joint should be visible.
3. Center and collimate further, if possible.
4. Expose.

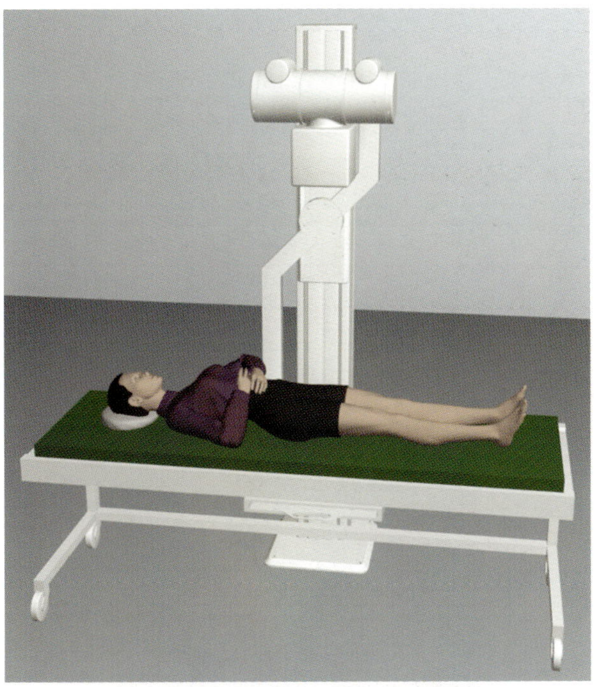

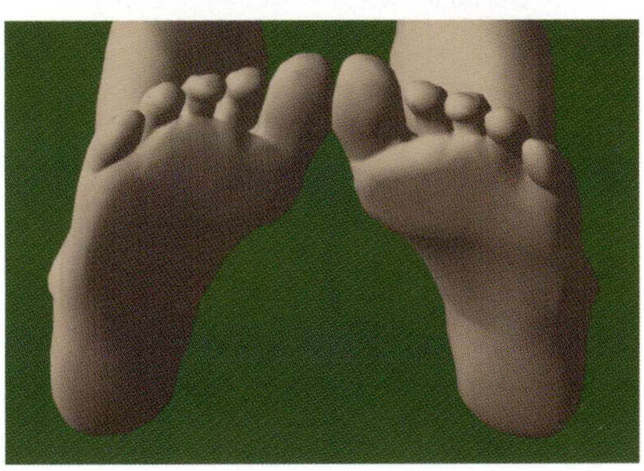

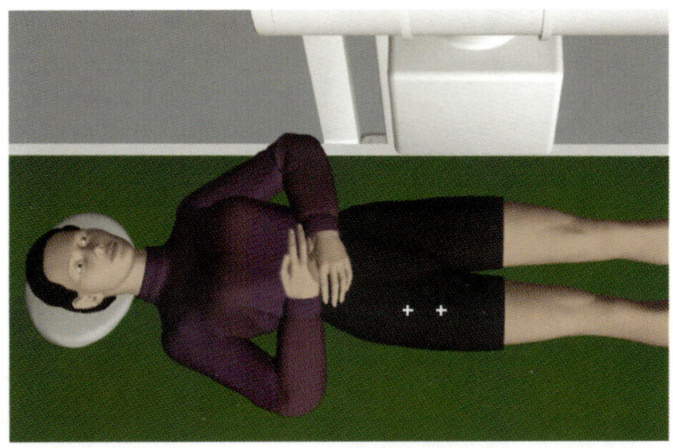

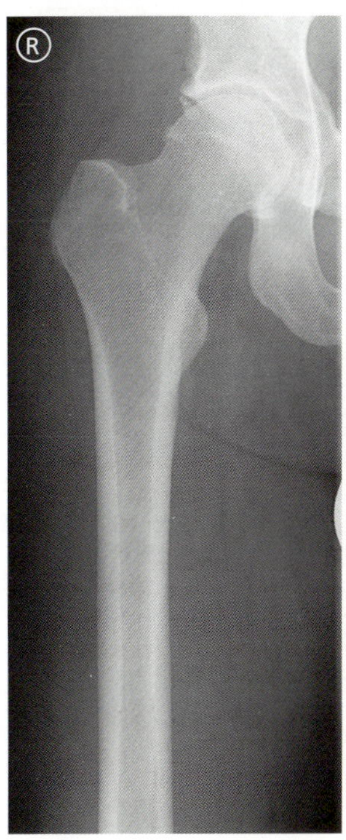

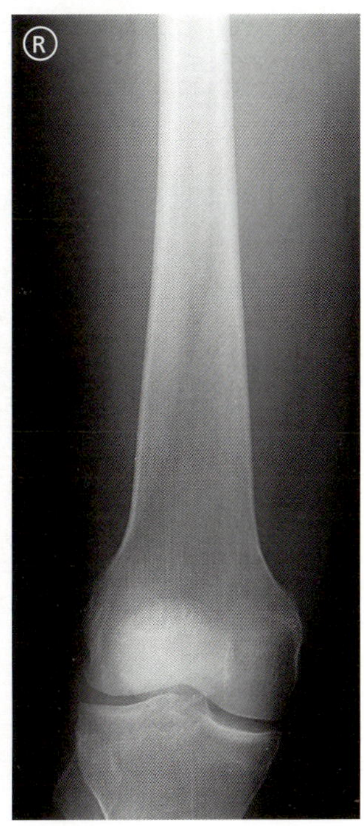

Hip and/or knee joint should be visible

FEMUR LATERAL **Lying on the side** BASIC

After injury, see LEG 8

Cassette speed
Cassette with screen-film combination, nominal speed 200/400 in the cassette holder. For a CHILD, cassette **on** the table

Cassette size
18×43 cm (7×17 inches)
24×30 cm (10×12 inches) for a child
Use a **R**ight or **L**eft marker

Exposure values	mAs	
70 **kV**	"blue" system 200	"green" system 400
Average	50	25
Range	32–100	16–40
Child 53 **kV**	"blue" system 200	"green" system 400/250
Range	3.2–8	2.5–6.3

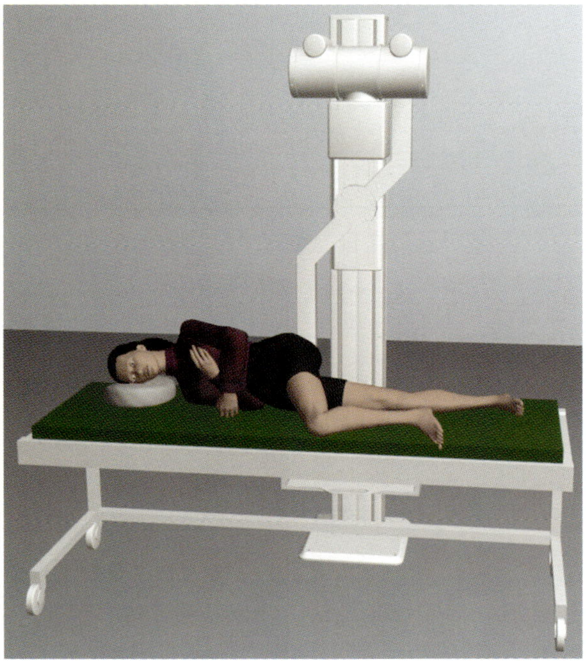

1. Bring in the patient, put the cassette in the cassette holder (on the table for a child). Collimate to the format.
2. Position the patient on the side to be examined with the leg straight.
3. Bend the other leg as shown.
4. Center and collimate further, if possible.
5. Expose.

For a lateral view of the upper end of the femur use LEG 4 or LEG 5.

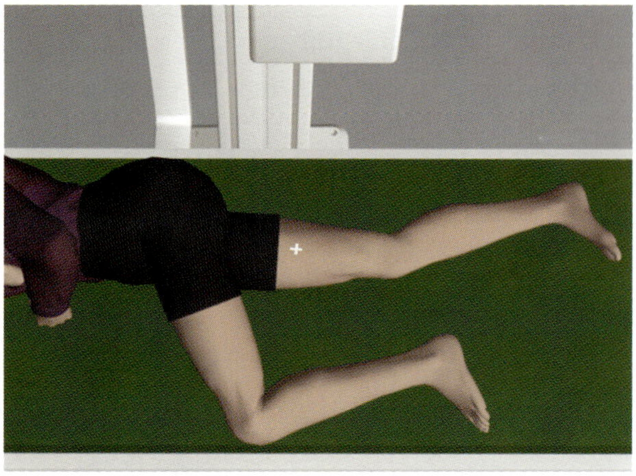

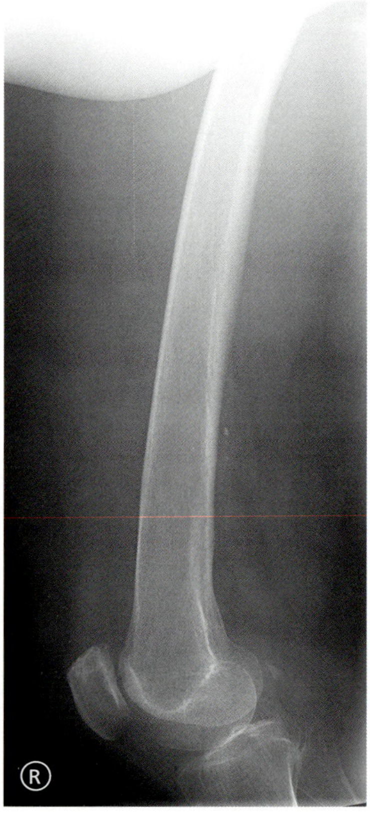

FEMUR LATERAL – after injury Supine – horizontal beam ADDITIONAL

Cassette speed
Cassette with screen-film combination, nominal speed 200/400 in the cassette holder.
For a CHILD, cassette **on** the table

Cassette size
18×43 cm (7×17 inches)
24×30 cm (10×12 inches) for a child
Use a **R**ight or **L**eft marker

Exposure values	mAs	
70 **kV**	"blue" system 200	"green" system 400
Average	50	25
Range	32–100	16–40
Child 53 **kV**	"blue" system 200	"green" system 400/250
Range	3.2–8	2.5–6.3

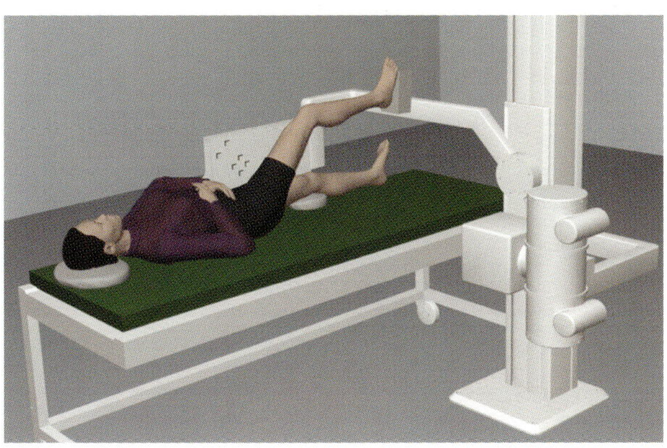

1. Bring in the patient, put the cassette in the cassette holder (on the table for a child). Collimate to the format.
2. Position the patient with the leg to be examined close to the cassette holder (cassette supported by a foam pad).
3. Bend and support the other leg as shown.
4. Center and collimate further, if possible. Make sure the knee joint is visible on the film.
5. Expose.

For a lateral view of the upper end of the femur use LEG 4 or LEG 5.

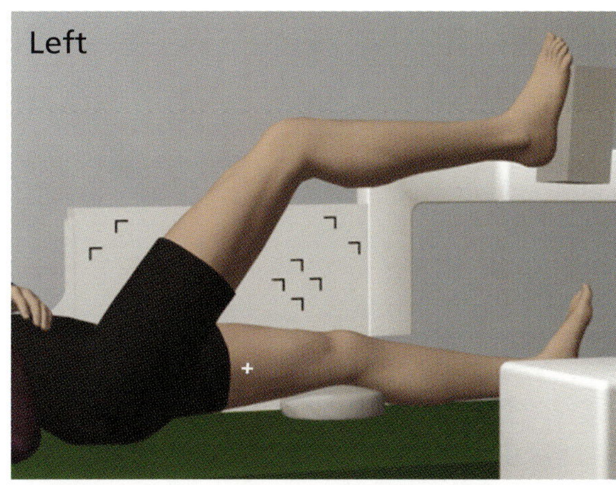

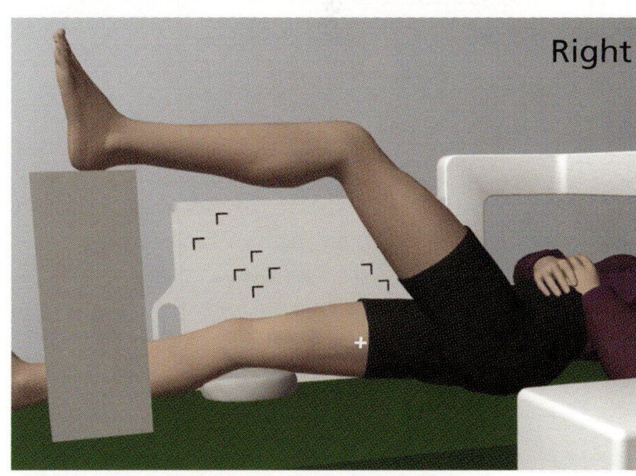

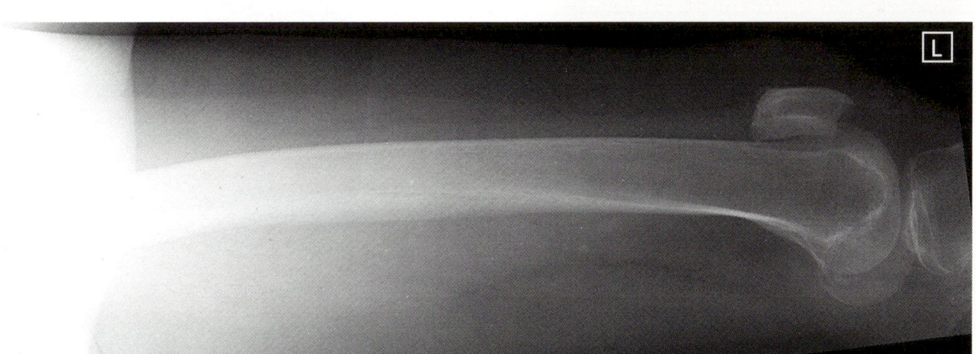

KNEE AP Supine BASIC

Cassette speed
Cassette with screen-film combination, nominal speed 50/100 on the table

Cassette size
18×24 cm (8×10 inches)
Use a **R**ight or **L**eft marker

Exposure values	mAs	
53 **kV**	"blue" system 50	"green" system 100/63
Average	50	40
Range	25–80	20–63

1. Bring in the patient, put the cassette on the table. Collimate to that format.
2. Position the patient. If possible, rotate the foot slightly inwards and steady it with a sandbag.
3. Center and collimate further, if possible.
4. Expose. Do knee lateral (LEG 10 or LEG 11) at the same time.

To find small fractures ADDITIONAL OBLIQUE VIEWS (45° rotation) may be ordered by the doctor when AP and LATERAL views have been valued.

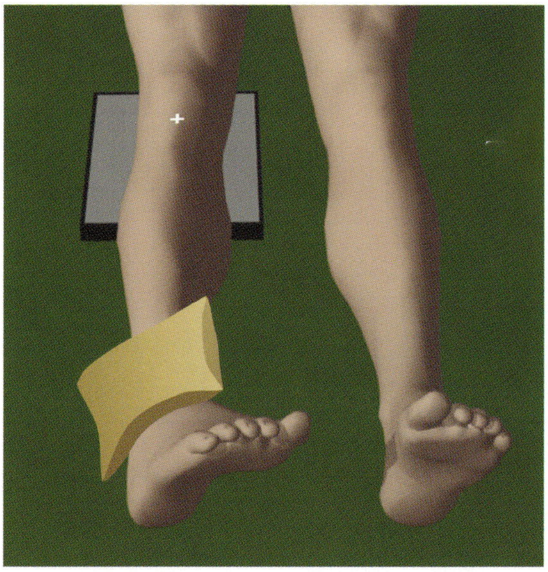

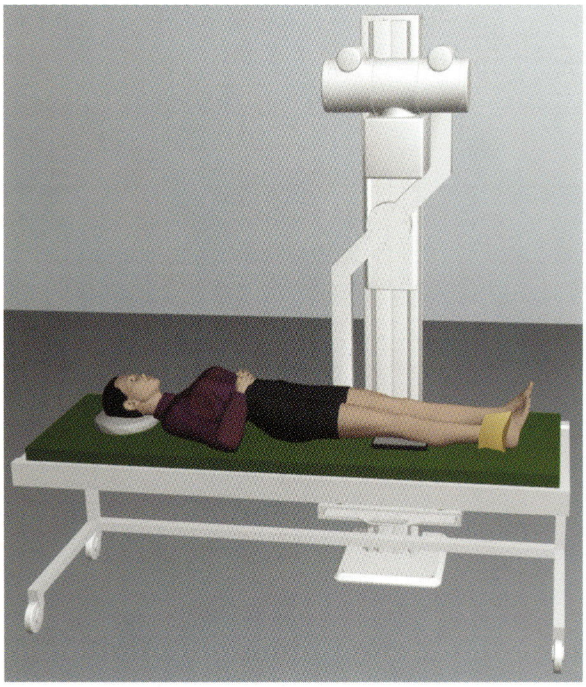

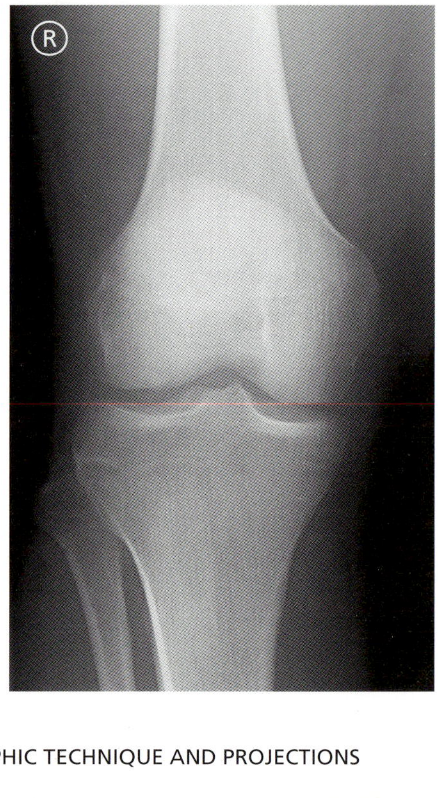

KNEE LATERAL Lying on the side BASIC

After injury, see LEG 11

Cassette speed
Cassette with screen-film combination, nominal speed 50/100 on the table

Cassette size
18×24 cm (8×10 inches)
Use a **R**ight or **L**eft marker

Exposure values	mAs	
53 **kV**	"blue" system 50	"green" system 100/63
Average	50	40
Range	25–80	20–63

1. Bring in the patient, put the cassette on the table. Collimate to that format.
2. Position the patient. Place the patient on the side to be examined with slightly bent knee. Support with a pad under the lower leg. Bend the other knee more and let it rest on the table.
3. Center and collimate further, if possible.
4. Expose.

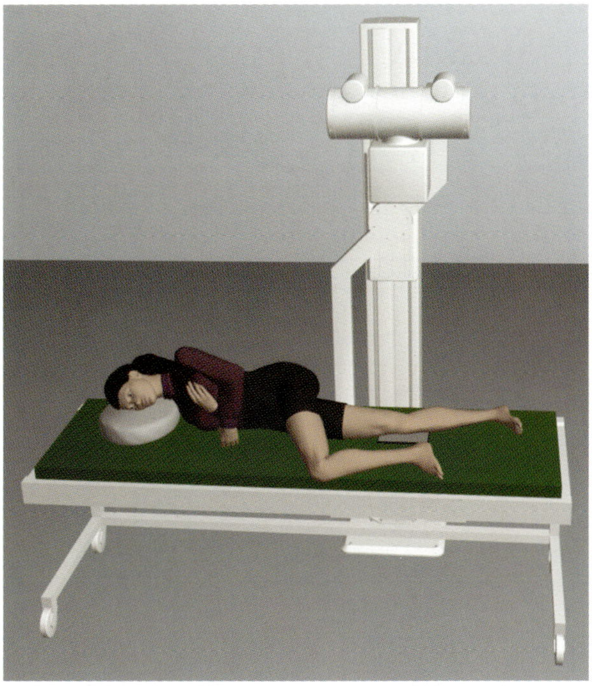

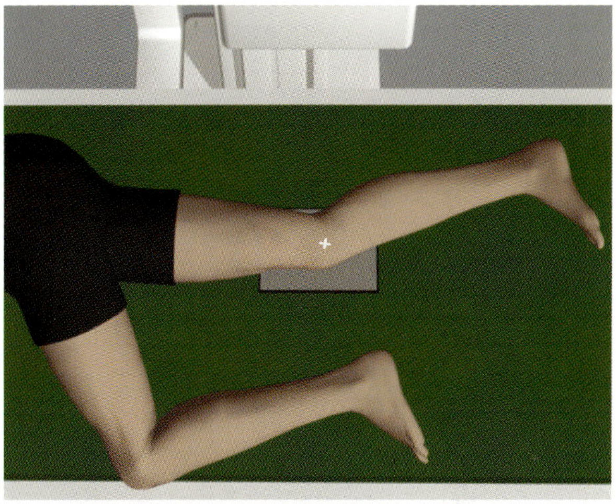

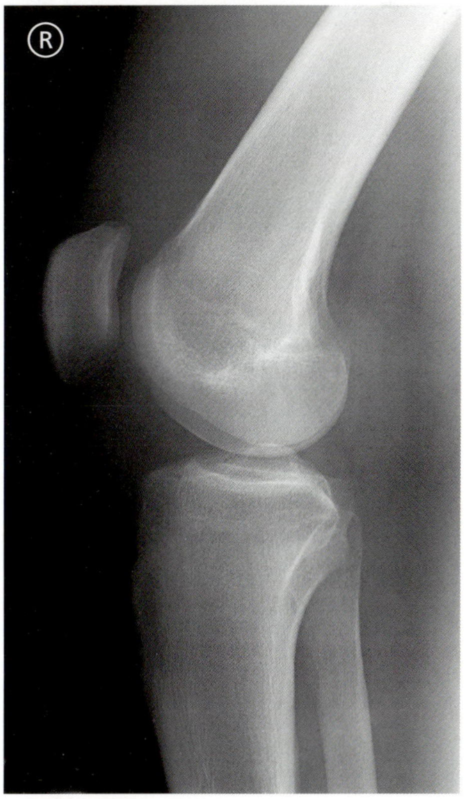

KNEE LATERAL – after injury Supine – horizontal beam ADDITIONAL

Cassette speed
Cassette with screen-film combination, nominal speed 50/100 on the table

Cassette size
18×24 cm (8×10 inches)
Use a **R**ight or **L**eft marker

Exposure values	mAs	
53 **kV**	"blue" system 50	"green" system 100/63
Average	50	40
Range	25–80	20–63

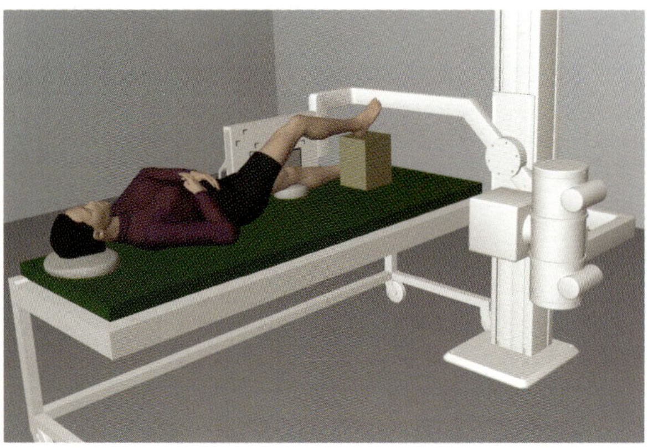

1. Bring in the patient, put the cassette on the table. Support the cassette by the side of the casette holder. Collimate to that format.
2. Position the patient with the cassette close to the leg to be examined. The cassette could be supported from the rear by a foam pad.
3. Bend and support the normal leg as shown.
4. Center and collimate further.
5. Expose.

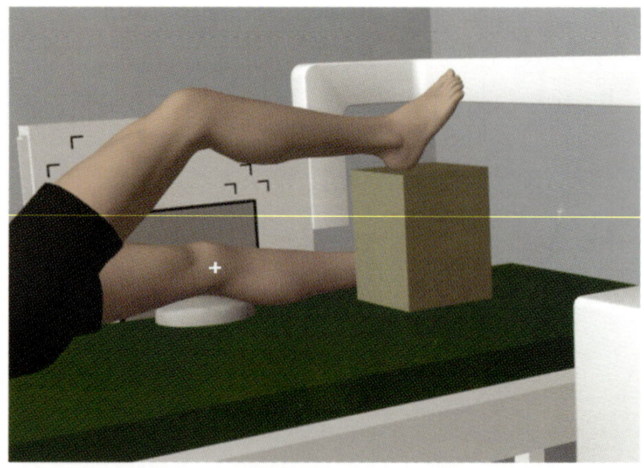

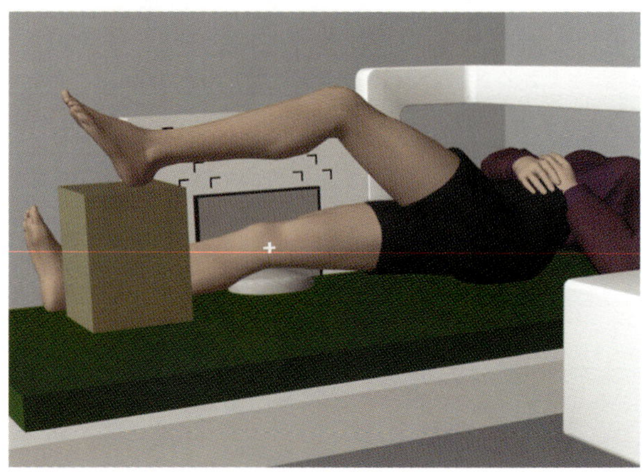

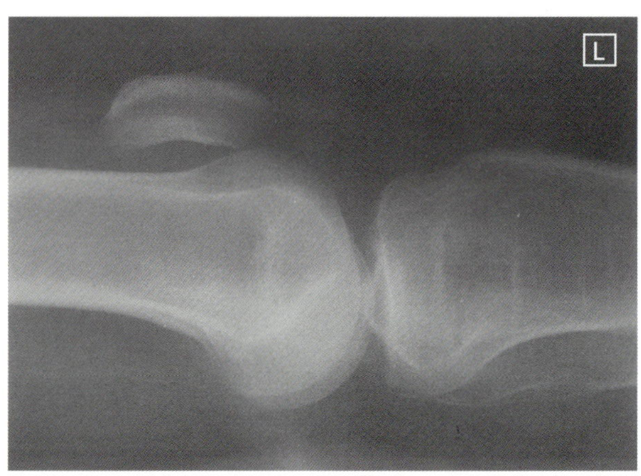

KNEE INTERCONDYLAR SPACE Supine – vertical beam angled 30° as shown

ADDITIONAL

Cassette speed
Cassette with screen-film combination, nominal speed 50/100 on the table on a support

Cassette size
18×24 cm (8×10 inches)
Use a **R**ight or **L**eft marker

Exposure values	mAs	
53 **kV**	"blue" system 50	"green" system 100/63
Average	40	32
Range	20–63	16–50

1. Bring in the patient. Place the cassette under the knee on a firm support 12–15 cm high as shown. Collimate to that format.
2. Position the patient with the cassette close to the leg to be examined.
3. Center and collimate further, if possible.
4. Expose.

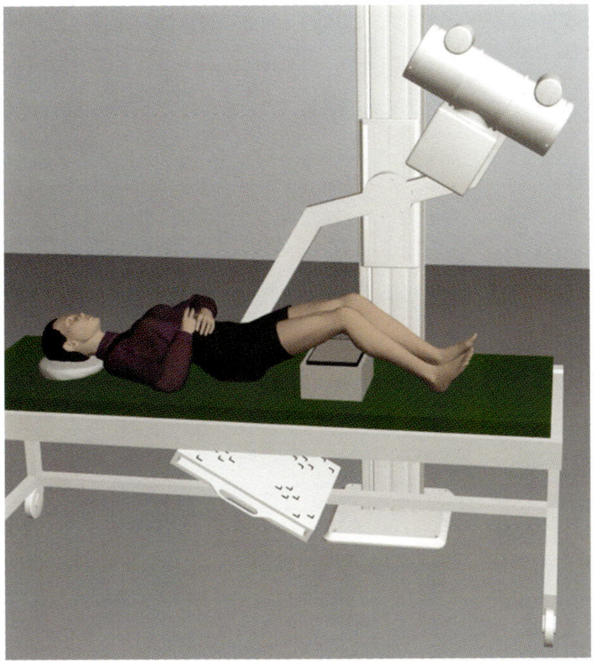

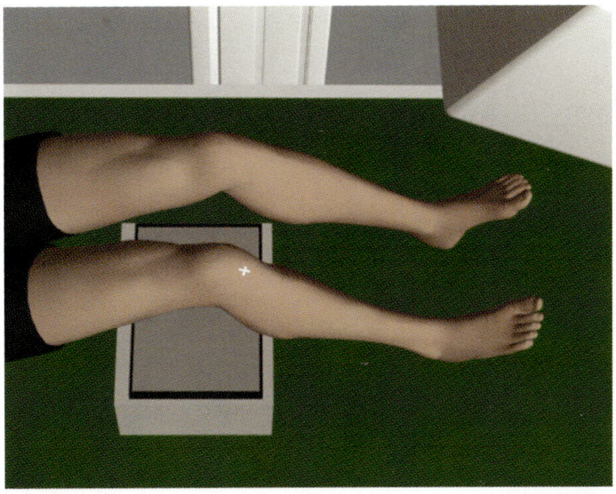

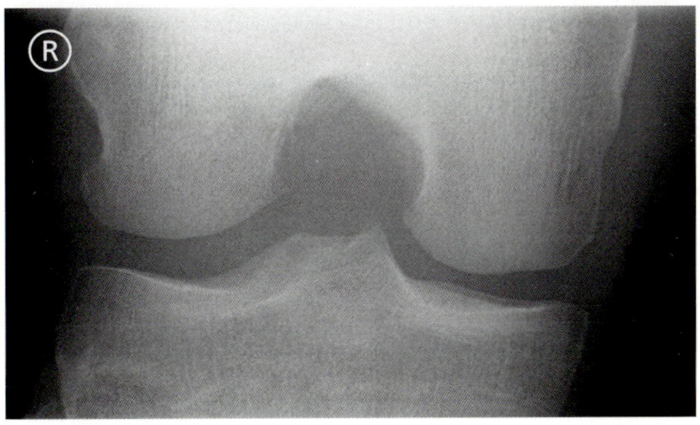

PATELLA AXIAL **Standing** ADDITIONAL

Cassette speed
Cassette with screen-film combination, nominal speed 50/100 on the casette holder on a support

Cassette size
18×24 cm (8×10 inches)
Use a **R**ight or **L**eft marker

Exposure values	mAs	
53 **kV**	"blue" system 50	"green" system 100/63
Average	32	25
Range	16–50	12.5–40

1. Bring in the patient. Place the cassette on top of the cassette holder on an about 25 cm high support as shown. Collimate to that format.
2. Position the patient with the cassette close to the leg to be examined.
3. Center and collimate further.
4. Expose.

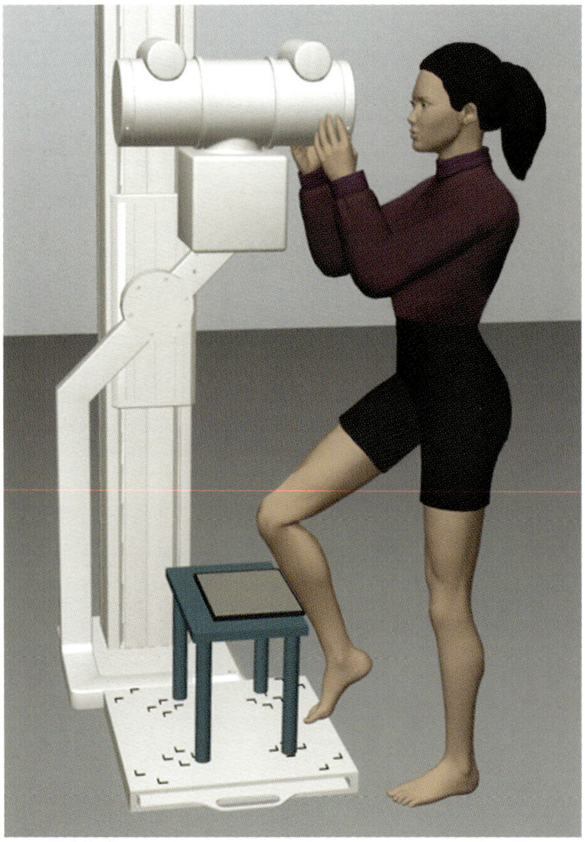

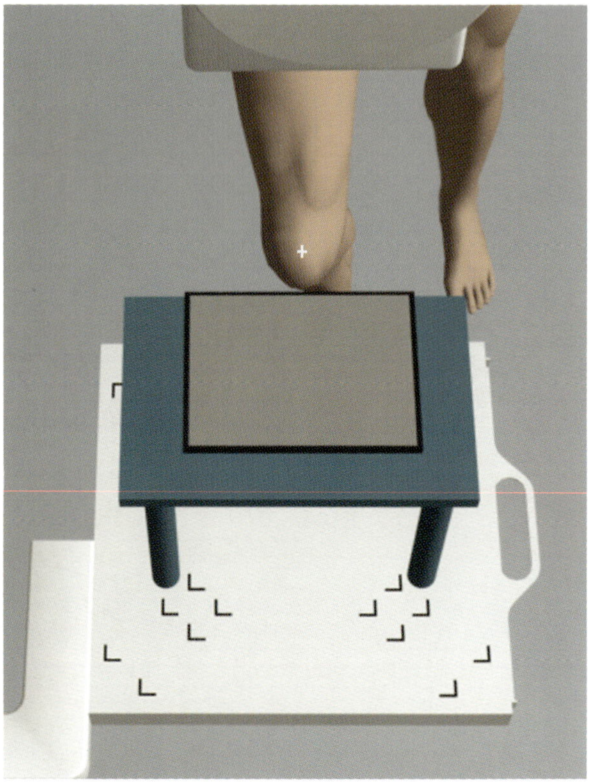

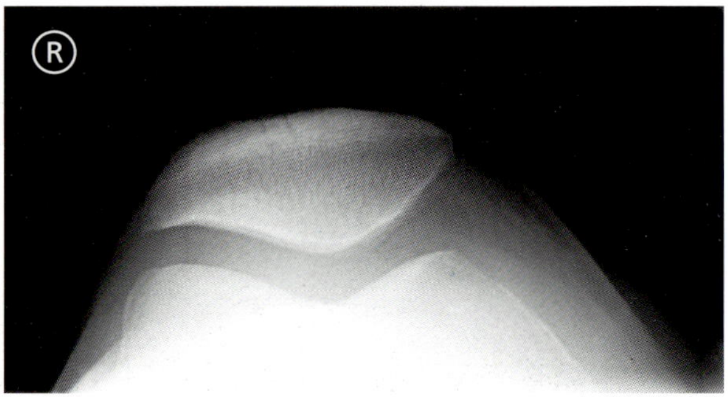

LOWER LEG AP Supine BASIC

Cassette speed
Cassette with screen-film combination, nominal speed 50/100 on the table

Cassette size
18×43 cm (7×17 inches)
35×43 cm (14×17 inches)
Use a **R**ight or **L**eft marker

Exposure values	mAs (average)	
53 **kV**	"blue" system 50	"green" system 100 /63
Including knee	40	32
Including ankle	25	20

1. Bring in the patient, put the cassette on the table. Collimate to that format.
2. Position the patient. If possible, rotate the foot slightly inwards and steady it with a sandbag.
3. Center and collimate further, if possible. At least one joint should be shown on the film. If injured the joint nearest the injury is to be visible. If the leg is in plaster, increase the exposure as shown in page 123.
4. Expose. Do leg lateral (LEG 15 or LEG 16) at the same time.

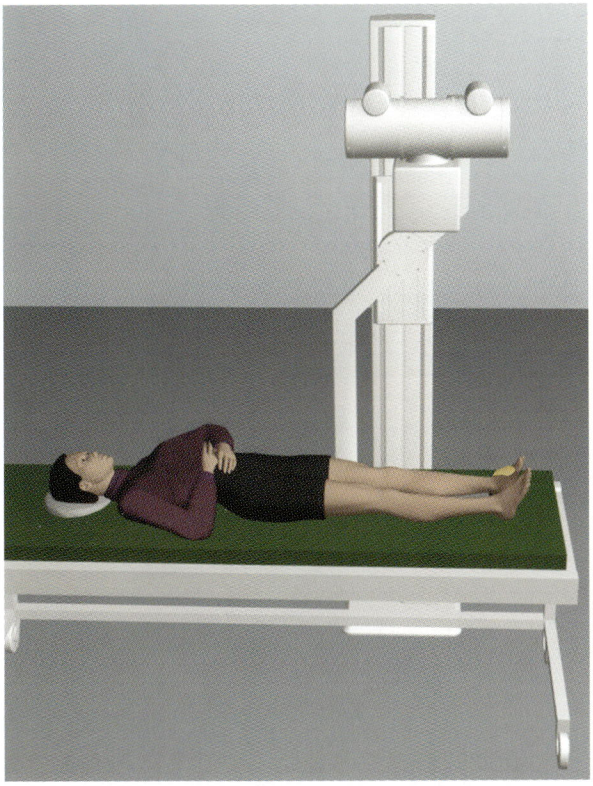

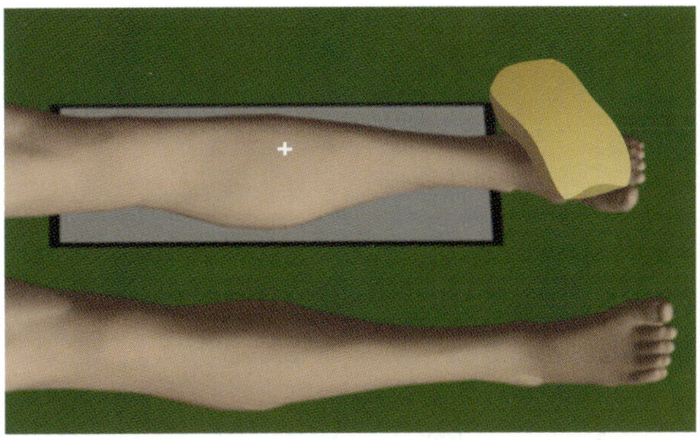

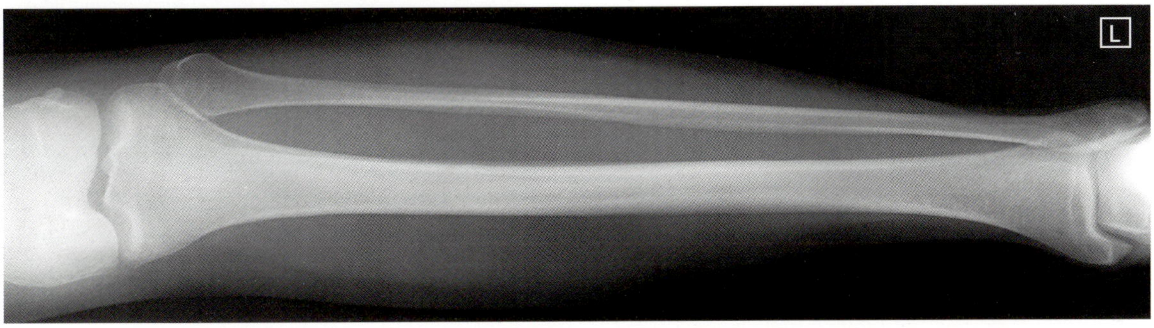

LOWER LEG LATERAL Lying on the side BASIC

If a fracture is suspected, use LEG 16

Cassette speed
Cassette with screen-film combination, nominal speed 50/100 on the table

Cassette size
18×43 cm (7×17 inches)
35×43 cm (14×17 inches)
Use a **R**ight or **L**eft marker

Exposure values	**mAs** (average)	
53 **kV**	"blue" system 50	"green" system 100 /63
Including knee	40	32
Including ankle	25	20

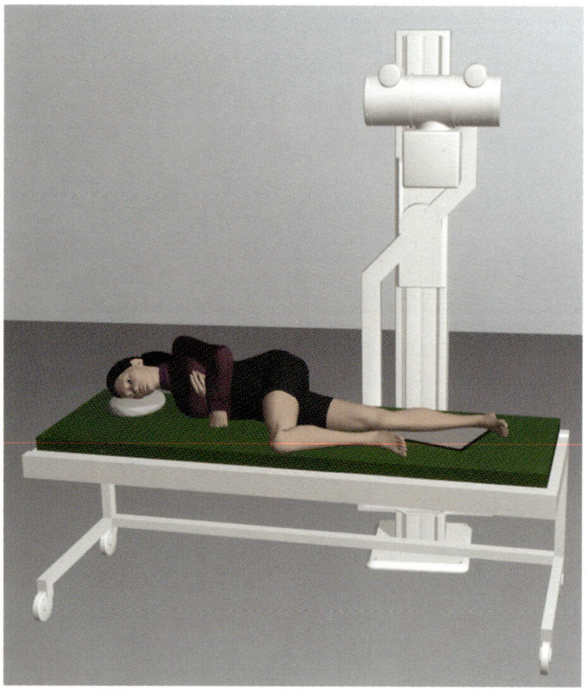

1. Bring in the patient, put the cassette on the table. Collimate to the format.
2. Place the patient on the side to be examined with slightly bent knee directly on the cassette. Bend the other knee more and let it rest on the table.
3. Center and collimate further. At least one joint should be visible on the film. If the leg is in plaster, increase the exposure as shown in page 123.
4. Expose.

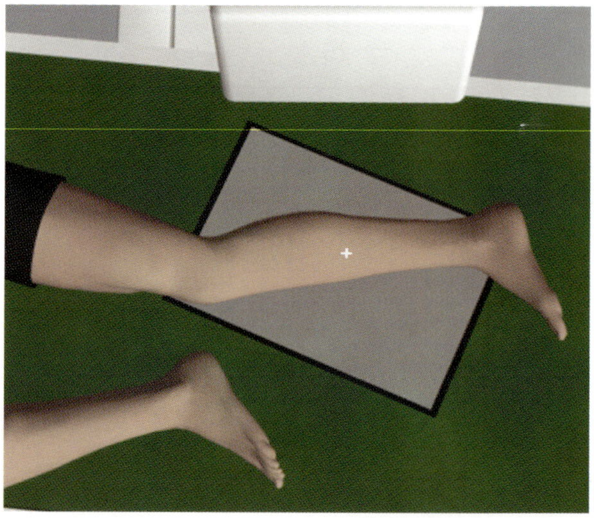

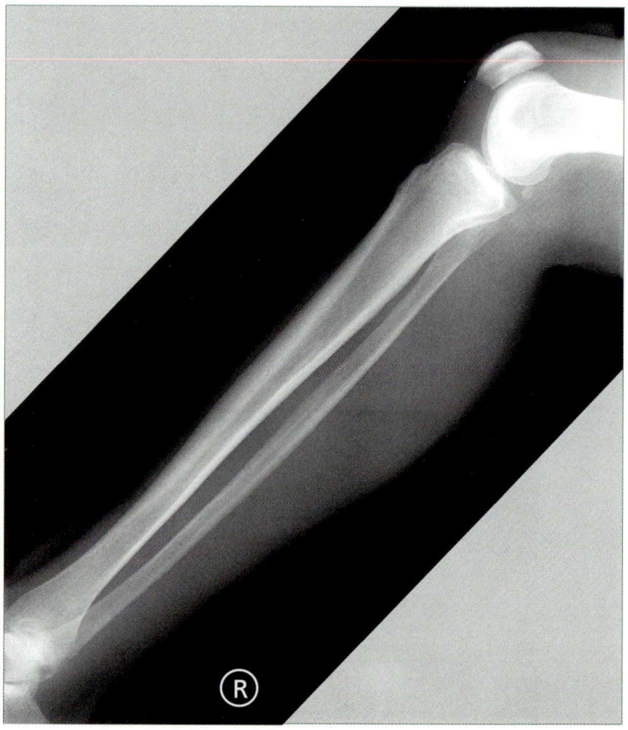

LOWER LEG LATERAL – after injury Supine – horizontal beam ADDITIONAL

Cassette speed
Cassette with screen-film combination, nominal speed 50/100 on the table

Cassette size
18×43 cm (7×17 inches)
Use a **R**ight or **L**eft marker

Exposure values	mAs (average)	
53 **kV**	"blue" system 50	"green" system 100 /63
Including knee	40	32
Including ankle	25	20

1. Bring in the patient, put the cassette on the table. Support the cassette by the side of the cassette holder.
2. Collimate to the format.
3. Position the patient. If possible, rotate the foot slightly inwards and steady it with a sandbag. If there are splints on the injured leg, leave them on. Bend the UNINJURED knee as shown and let it rest on the table.
4. Center and collimate further. At least one joint should be visible on the film. The joint nearest to the injury should be visible. If the leg is in plaster, increase the exposure as shown in page 123.
5. Expose.

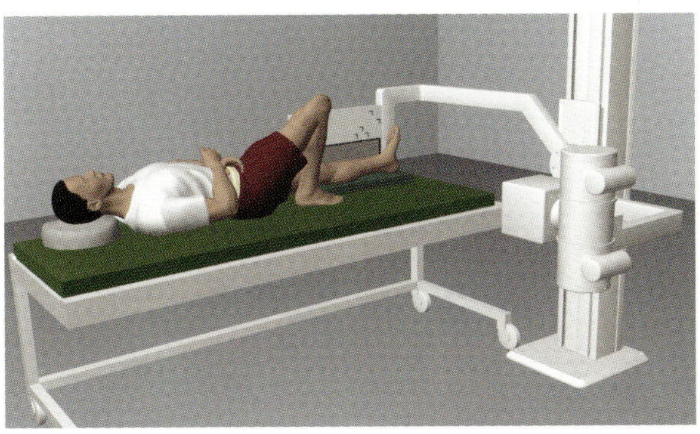

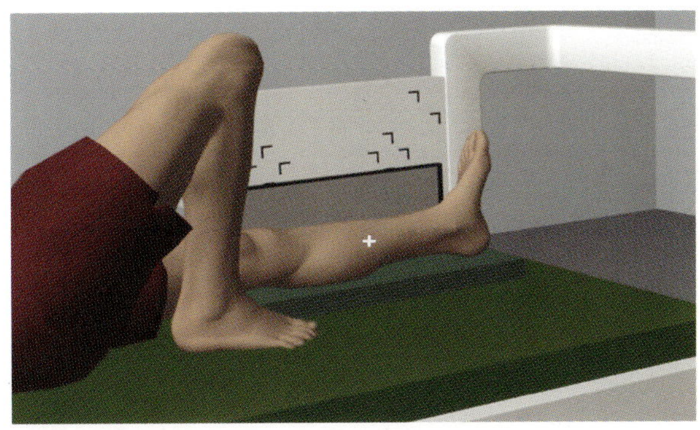

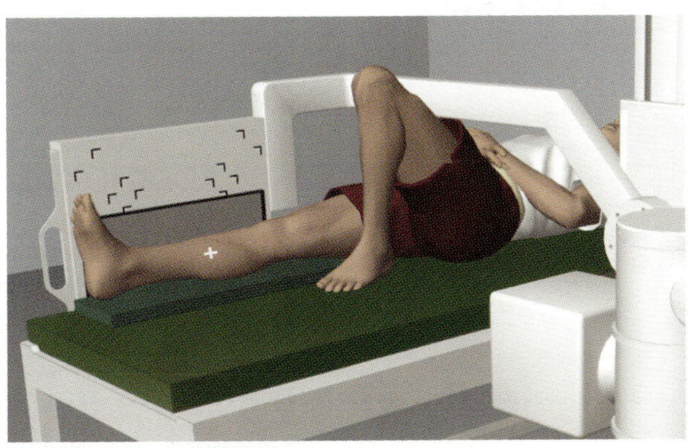

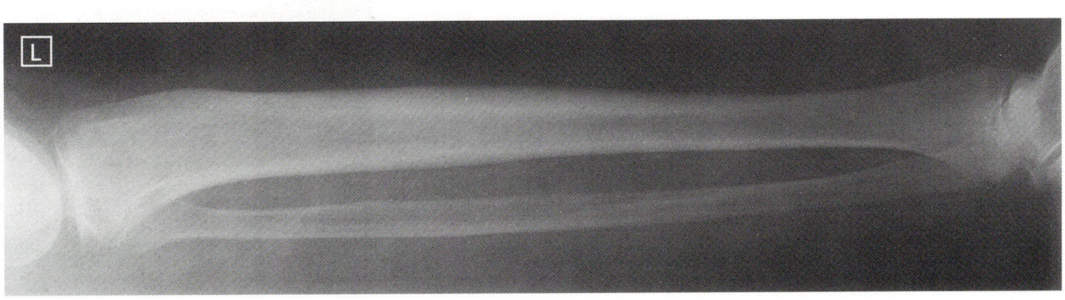

ANKLE JOINT INTERNAL OBLIQUE **Supine** BASIC
and **ANKLE JOINT AP** **Supine** ADDITIONAL

Cassette speed
Cassette with screen-film combination, nominal speed 50/100 on the table

Cassette size
18×24 cm (8×10 inches)
Use a **R**ight or **L**eft marker

Exposure values	mAs	
53 kV	"blue" system 50	"green" system 100 /63
Average	25	20
Range	16–50	12.5–40

1. Bring in the patient, put the cassette on the table. Collimate to that format.
2. Position the patient, sitting or lying down. For internal oblique rest the patients heel on the cassette and turn the foot inwards at a 15° angle. For AP (only when requested by the doctor) keep the foot straight up.
3. Center and collimate further.
4. Expose.

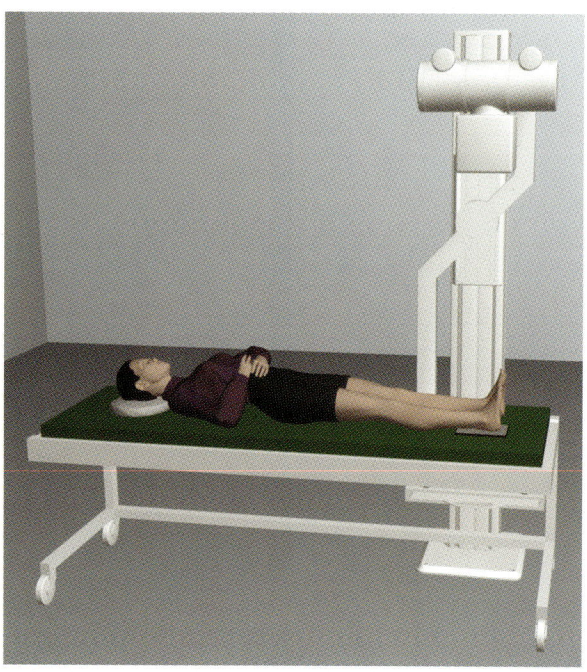

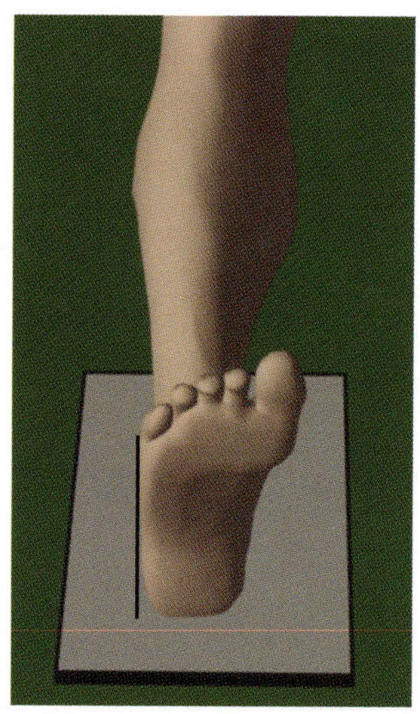

AP
ADDITIONAL

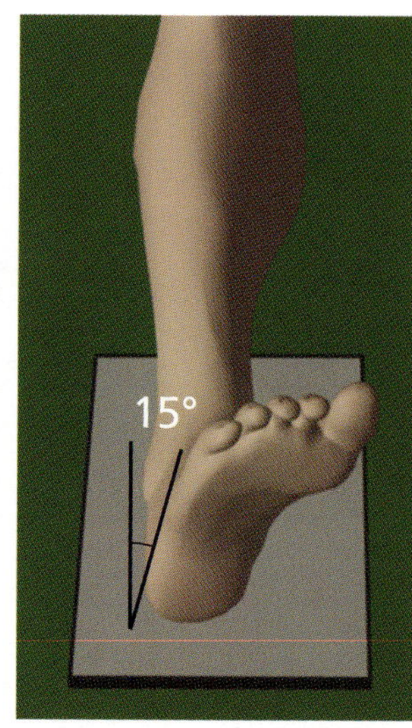

Internal oblique
BASIC

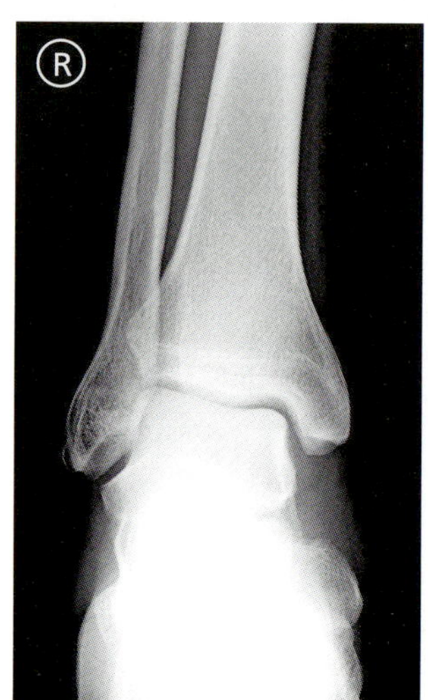

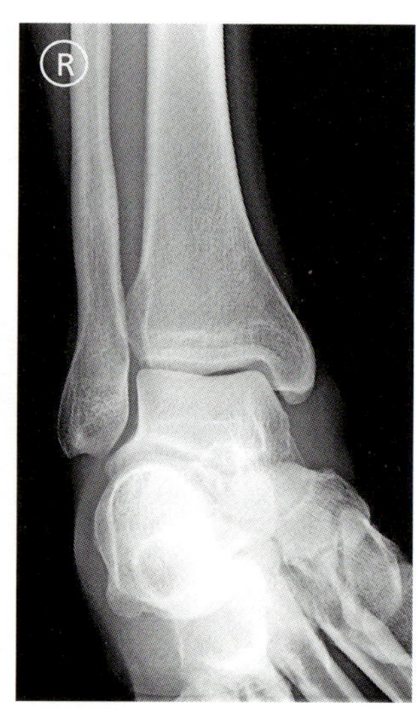

ANKLE JOINT LATERAL Supine BASIC and ANKLE JOINT EXTERNAL OBLIQUE Supine ADDITIONAL

Cassette speed
Cassette with screen-film combination, nominal speed 50/100 on the table

Cassette size
18×24 cm (8×10 inches)
Use a **R**ight or **L**eft marker

Exposure values	mAs	
53 **kV**	"blue" system 50	"green" system 50/100
Average	20/25	16/20
Range	16–50	12.5–40

1. Bring in the patient, put the cassette on the table. Collimate to the format.
2. Position the patient, sitting or lying down. For lateral, rotate the patient's leg outwards so that the foot rests against the cassette. For external oblique (only when requested by the doctor), rest the patients heel on the cassette and rotate outwards so that the foot is in 30° angle to the cassette.
3. Center and collimate further.
4. Expose.

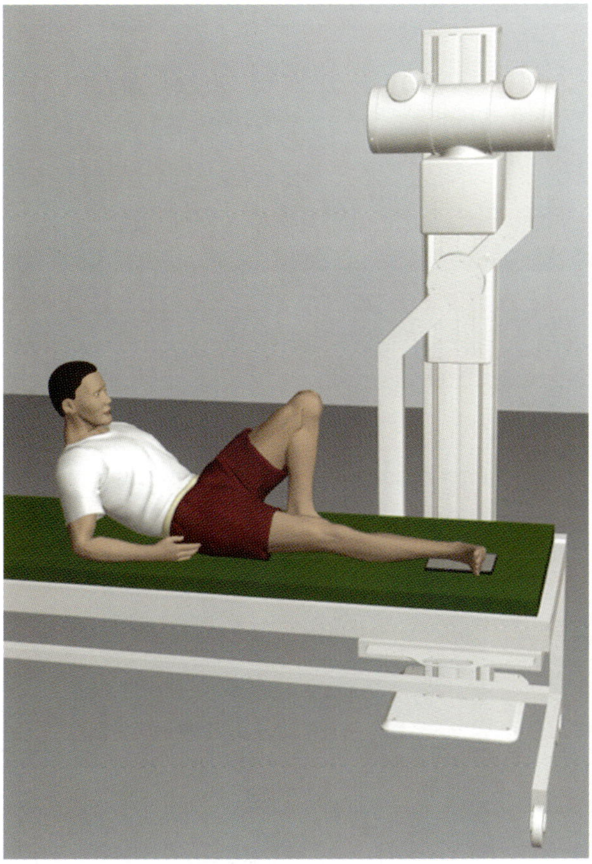

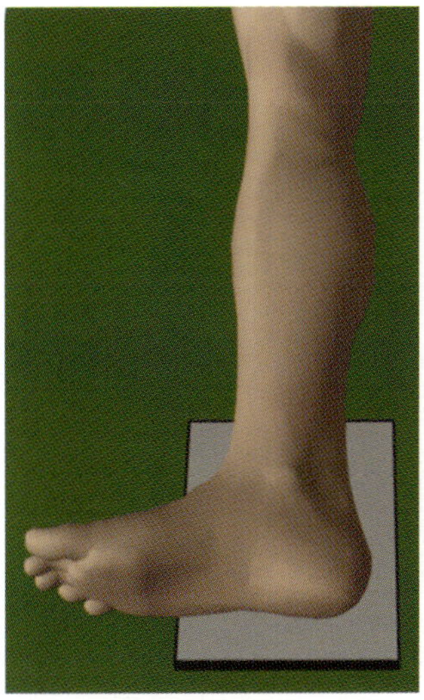

Lateral
BASIC

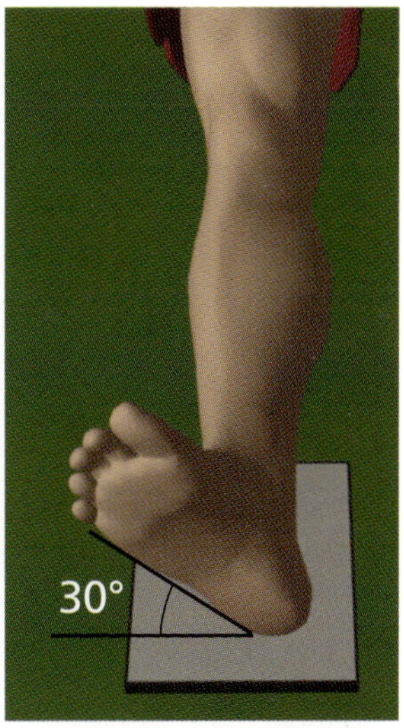

External oblique
ADDITIONAL

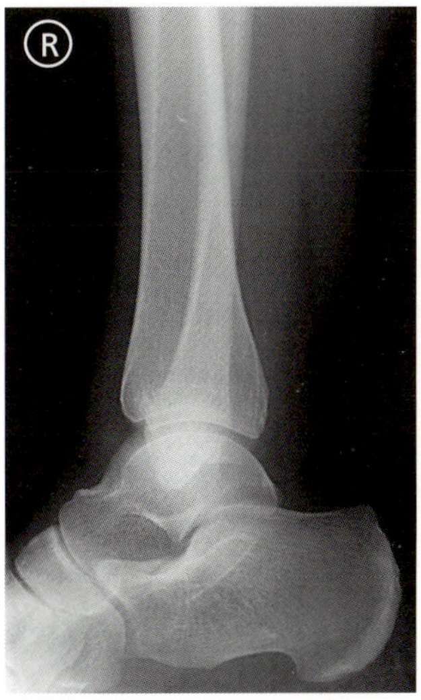

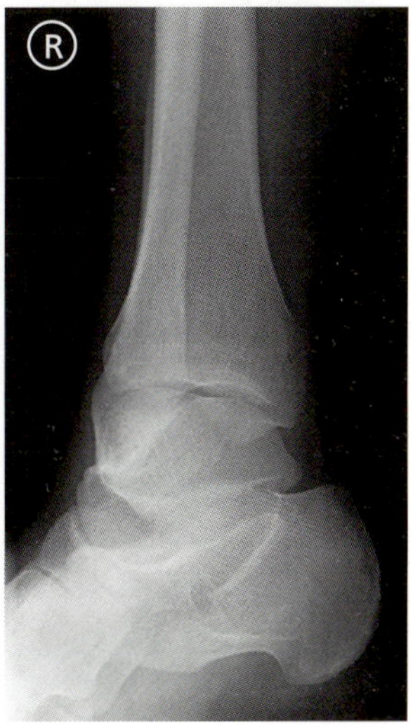

FOOT AP and TOES AP Supine – vertical beam angled 10° as shown BASIC

Cassette speed
Cassette with screen-film combination, nominal speed 50/100 on the table

Cassette size
18×24 cm (8×10 inches)
Use a **R**ight or **L**eft marker

Exposure values	mAs	
46 **kV**	"blue" system 50	"green" system 100/50
Average	25	25
Range	20–64	20–64
Toes	10	10

1. Bring in the patient, put the cassette on the table. Collimate to the format.
2. Position the patient, sitting or lying down. The foot rests flat on the cassette with the patients leg bent.
   Center and collimate further.
3. Use half of the mAs values for toes only.
4. Expose.

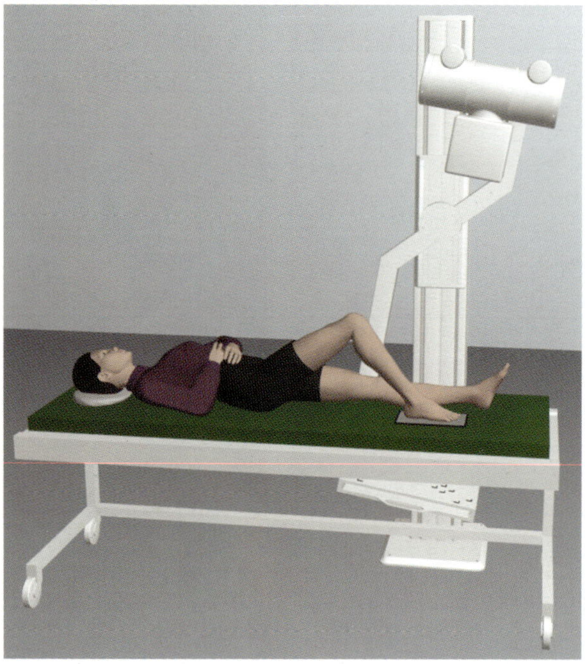

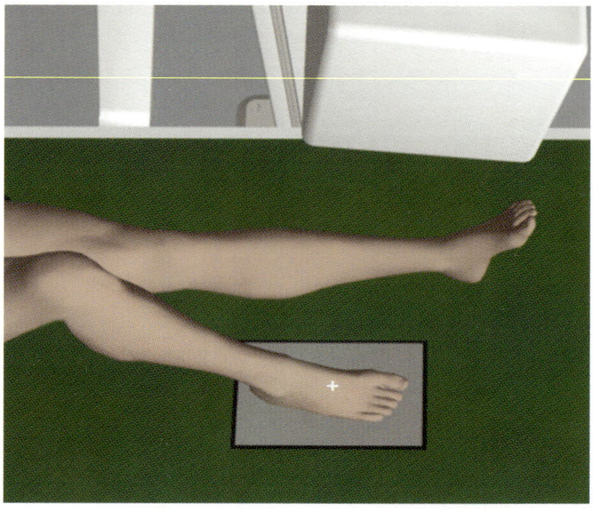

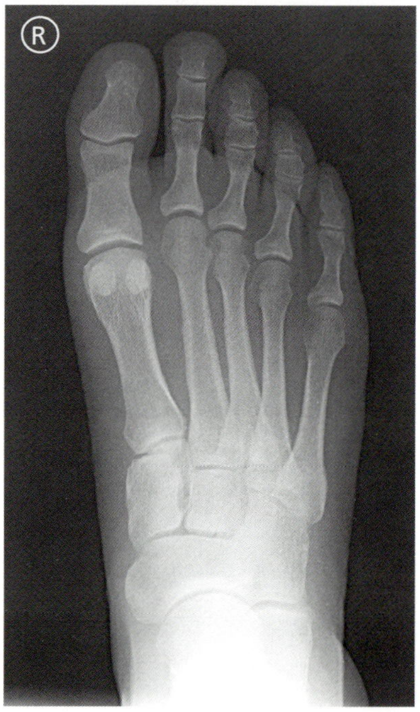

FOOT LATERAL Lying on the side ADDITIONAL

Cassette speed
Cassette with screen-film combination, nominal speed 50/100 on the table

Cassette size
18×24 cm (8×10 inches)
24×30 cm (10×12 inches)
Use a **R**ight or **L**eft marker

Exposure values	mAs	
46 **kV**	"blue" system 50	"green" system 100/50
Average	25	25
Range	20–64	20–64

1. Bring in the patient, put the cassette, small for a small foot, large for a large foot on the table. Collimate to the format.
2. Position the patient, lying down on the side to be examined with the knees bent as shown. Center and collimate further.
3. Expose.

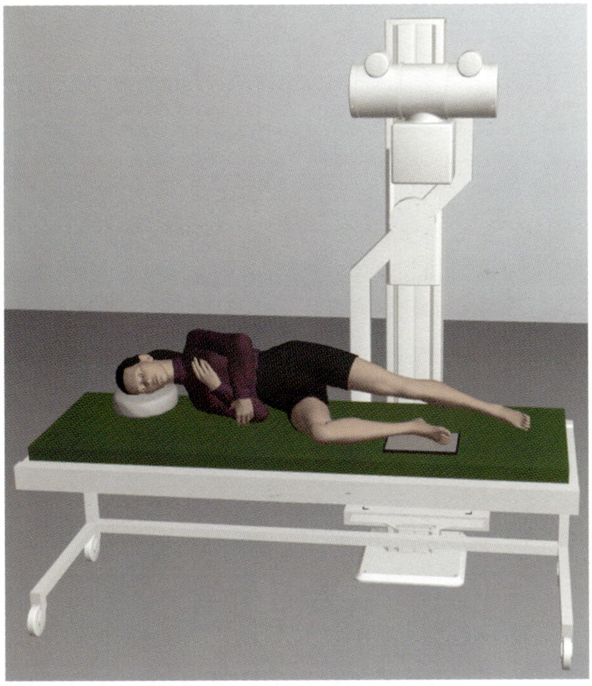

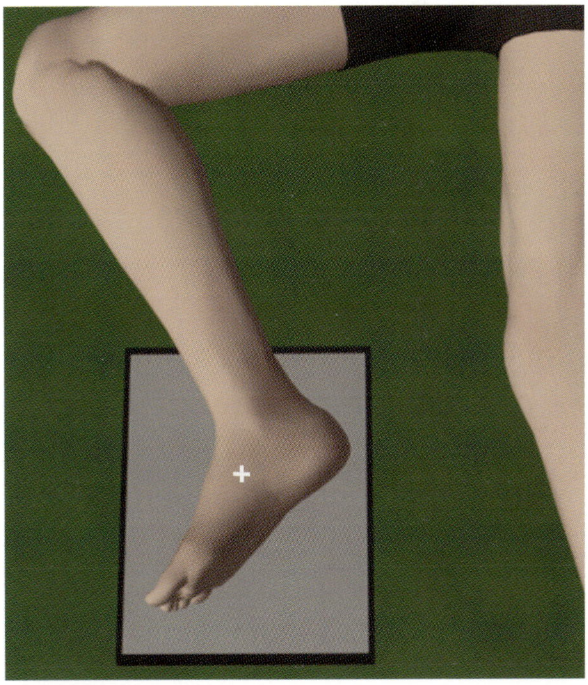

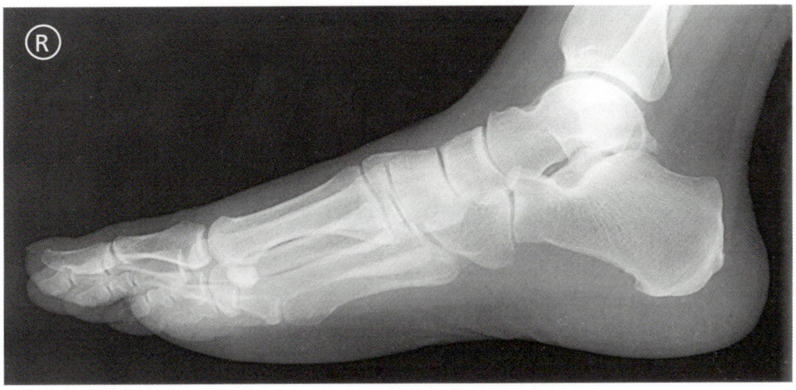

FOOT PA OBLIQUE Prone BASIC

Cassette speed
Cassette with screen-film combination, nominal speed 50/100 on the table

Cassette size
18×24 cm (8×10 inches)
24×30 cm (10×12 inches)
Use a **R**ight or **L**eft marker

Exposure values	mAs	
46 **kV**	"blue" system 50	"green" system 100/50
Average	25	25
Range	20–64	20–64

1. Bring in the patient, put the cassette, small for a small foot, large for a very large foot, on the table. Collimate to the format.
2. Position the patient, lying prone on the table as shown. Center and collimate further.
3. Expose.

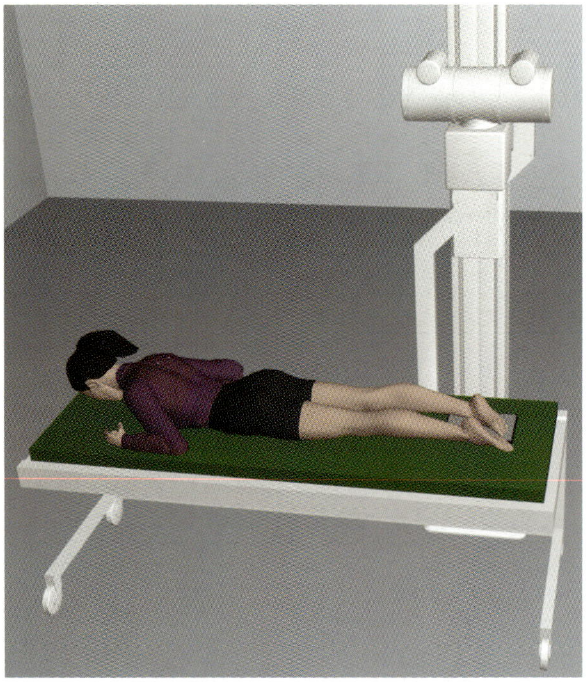

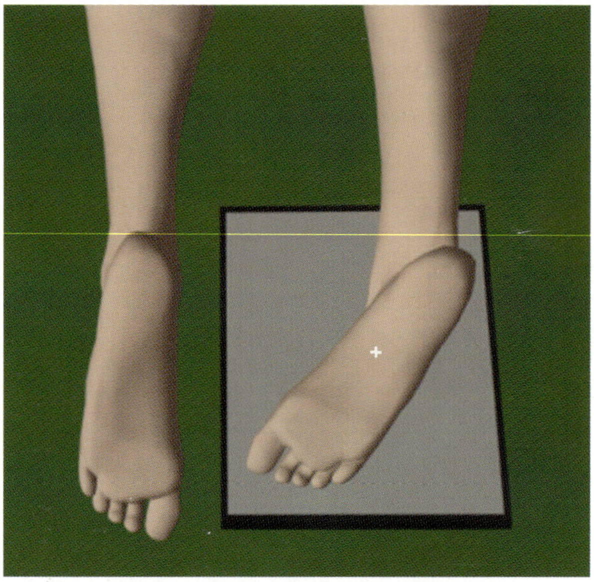

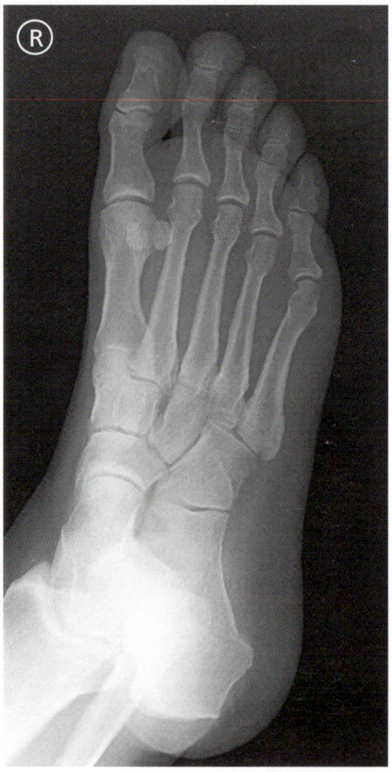

FOOT AP OBLIQUE   Sitting on the table – vertical beam angled 15° as shown

ADDITIONAL

Cassette speed
Cassette with screen-film combination, nominal speed 50/100 on the table

Cassette size
18x24 cm (7x9 inches)
24x30 cm (9x12 inches)
Use a **R**ight or **L**eft marker

Exposure values	mAs	
46 **kV**	"blue" system 50	"green" system 100/50
Average	25	25
Range	20–64	20–64

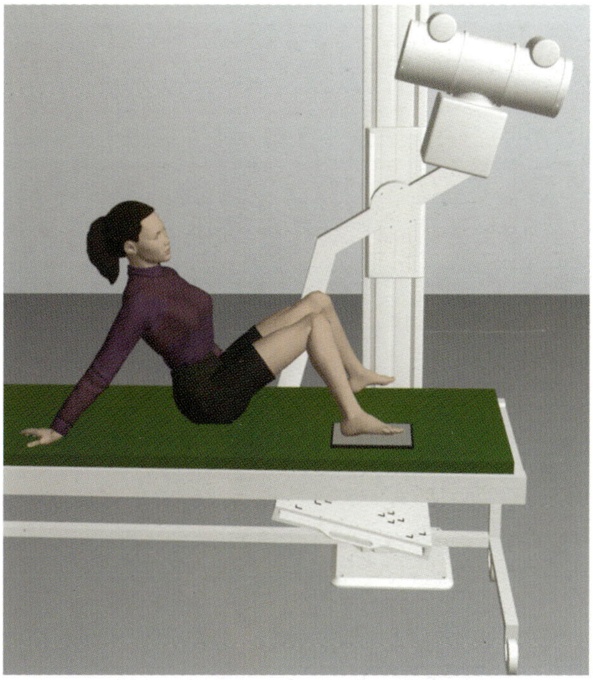

1. Bring in the patient, put the cassette, small for a small foot, large for a very large foot, on the table. Collimate to the format.
2. Position the patient, angle the foot as shown. Center and collimate further.
3. Expose.

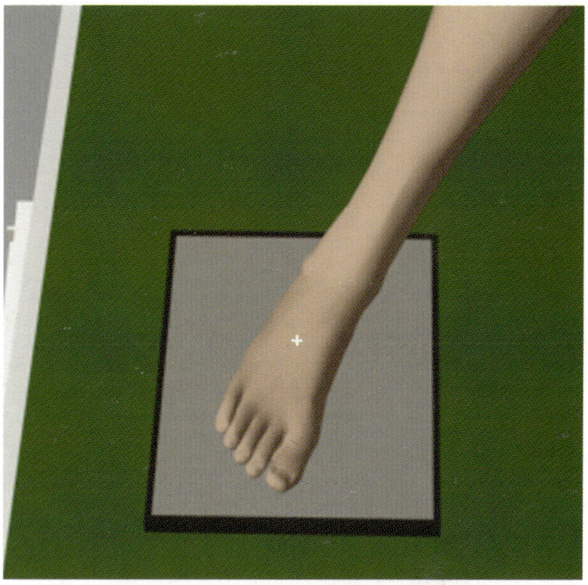

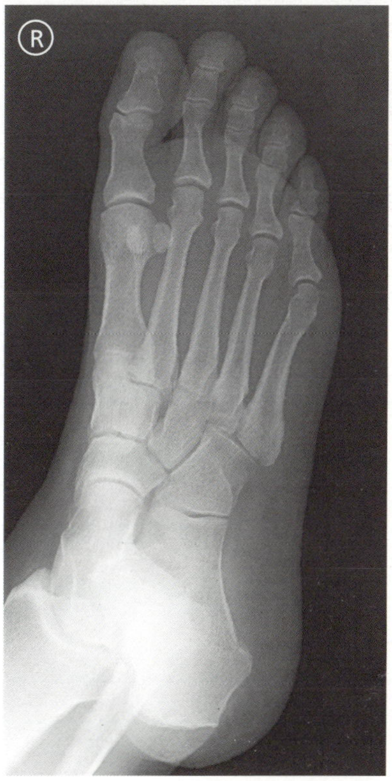

HEEL SEMIXIAL **Supine – vertical beam angled 30° as shown** BASIC

Lateral view, use LEG 18, but centre over the heel.

Cassette speed

Cassette with screen-film combination, nominal speed 50/100 on the table

Cassette size

18×24 cm (8×10 inches)

Use a **R**ight or **L**eft marker

Exposure values	mAs	
53 **kV**	"blue" system 50	"green" system 100/63
Average	25	20
Range	16–40	12.5–32

1. Bring in the patient, put the cassette on the table. Collimate to the format. Angle 30° as shown.
2. Position the patient; the foot should be pulled up as shown by means of a string held by the patient.
3. Center and collimate further.
4. When the patient is INJURED use either this position or that shown for LEG 24, whichever causes the least pain.
5. Expose.

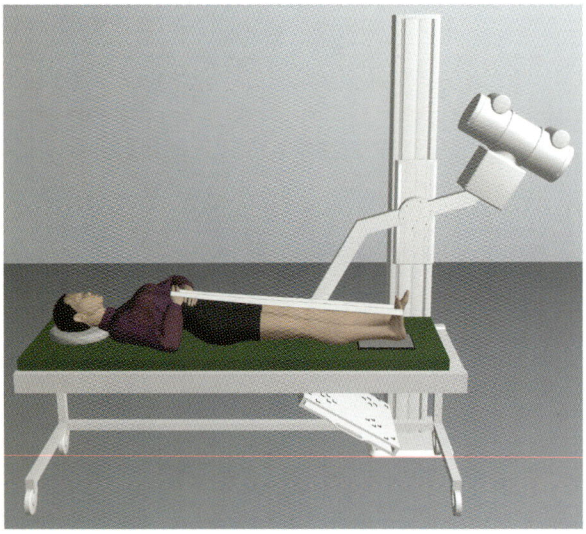

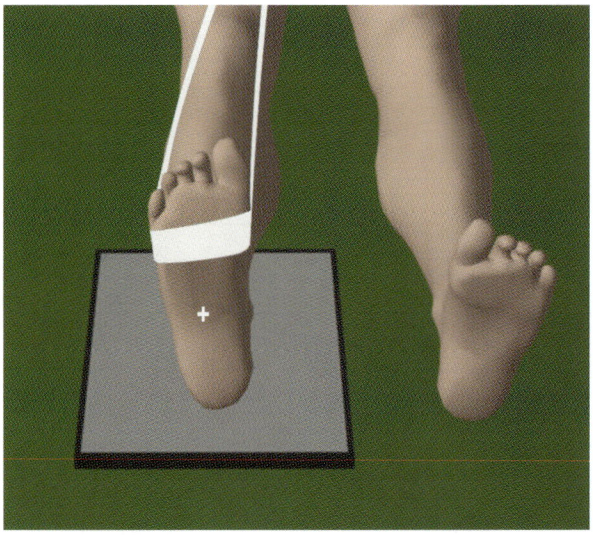

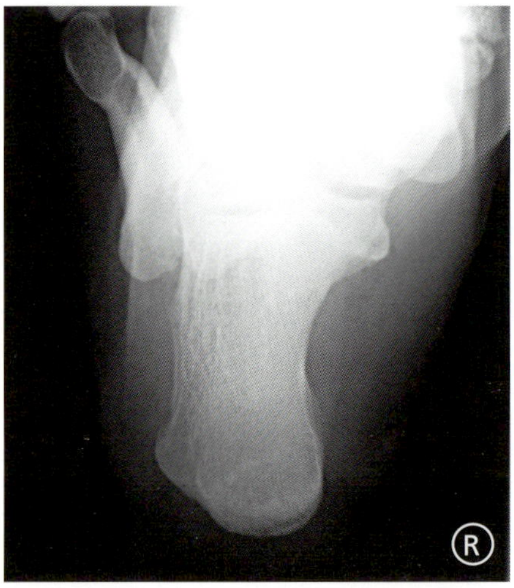

HEEL SEMIXIAL Prone – beam angled 60° as shown ADDITIONAL

Cassette speed
Cassette with screen-film combination, nominal speed 50/100 in the cassette holder

Cassette size
18×24 cm (8×10 inches)
Use a **R**ight or **L**eft marker

Exposure values	mAs	
70 **kV**	"blue" system 50	"green" system 100
Average	64	32
Range	40–100	20–50

1. Bring in the patient, put the cassette in the cassette holder. Collimate to the format. Angle 60° as shown.
2. Position the patient, prone, the toes against the cassette holder.
   Center and collimate further.
3. When the patient is INJURED use either this position or that shown for LEG 23, whichever causes the least pain.
4. Expose.

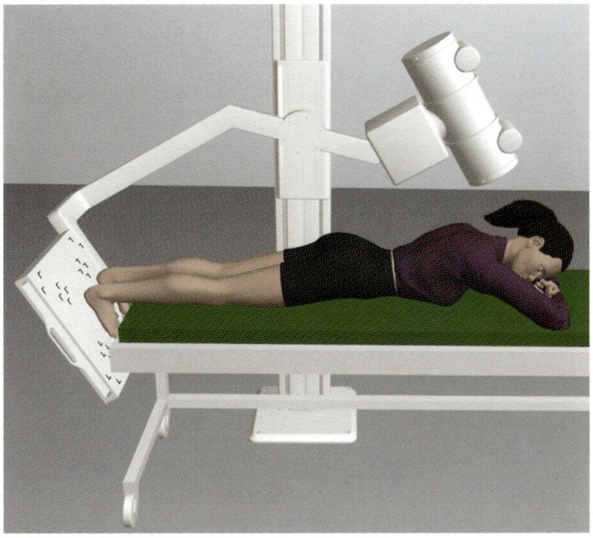

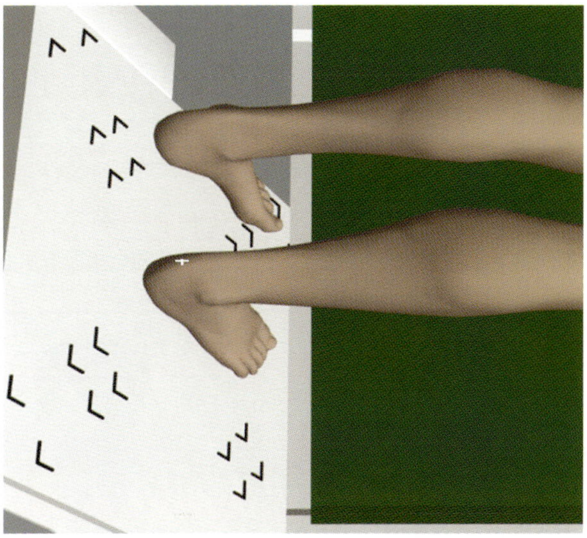

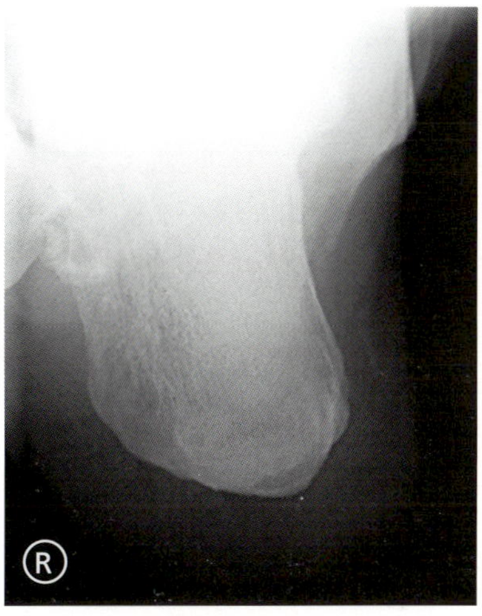

PELVIS AND HIP JOINTS AP Supine BASIC

Infants and small children

Cassette speed
Cassette with screen-film combination, nominal speed 200/400 on the cassette holder

Cassette size
18×24 cm (8×10 inches)
Use a **R**ight or **L**eft marker

Exposure values	mAs	
53 **kV**	"blue" system 200	"green" system 400/250
Average	6.3	5
Range	4–12.5	3.3–10

1. Bring in the patient, place the cassette on top of the cassette holder. Collimate to the format.
2. The child must be supported by the legs (knee joints) and either the arms or the body. Those supporting the child, preferably the PARENTS, MUST WEAR LEAD APRONS and, whenever possible, LEAD GLOVES.
3. Lie the child on its back on the cassette. Strech the legs. Centre a little above the pubic symphysis and collimate further.
4. Expose when the child is not moving.

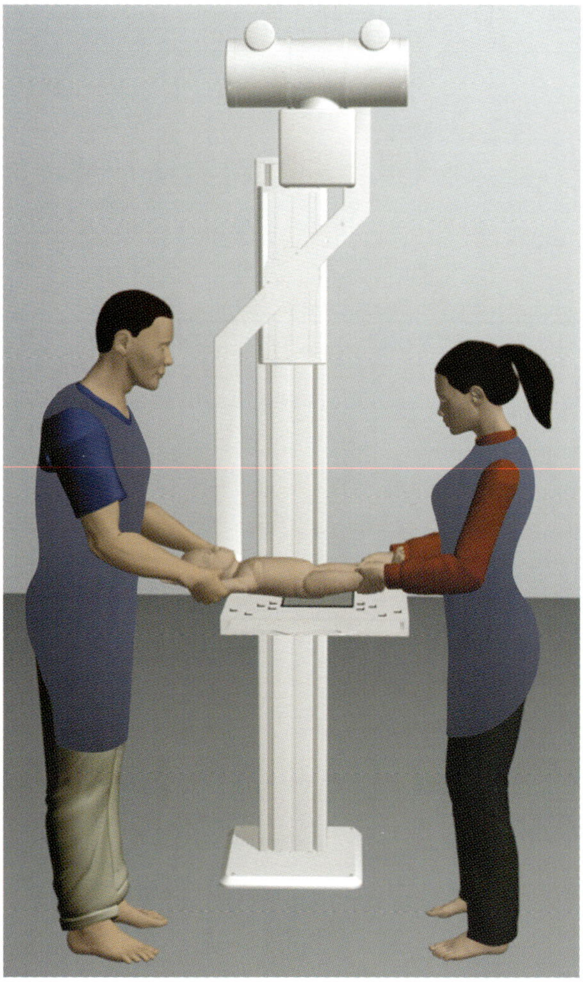

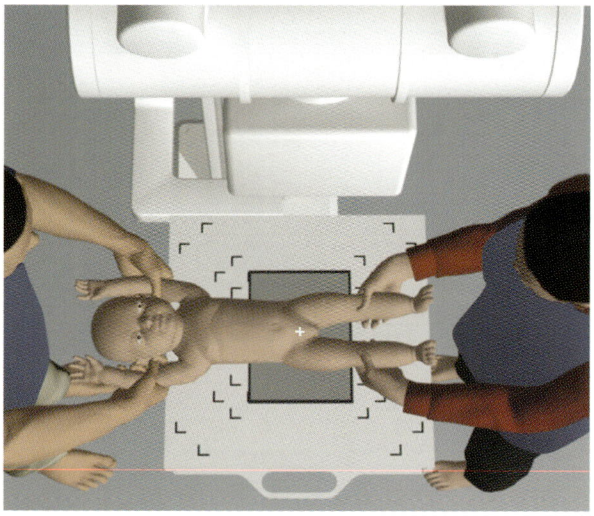

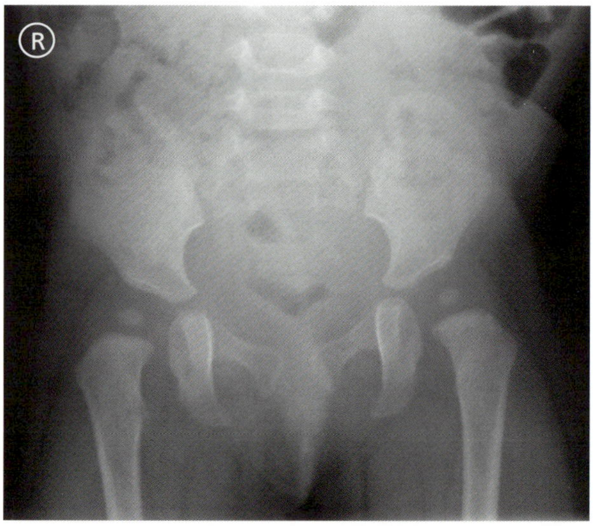

Comments

The persons holding the child must wear lead aprons and, if possible, lead gloves.

Film processing

Applying correct positioning, projections, exposure dates, etc., as described in the previous chapters is not enough to achieve a good end result of the radiographic examination. Correct and professional film processing is equally important.

The instructions in this chapter are valid both for automatic and manual film processing.

Automatic film processing

If an automatic film processing is used, it is important to follow the instructions that come with the machine. It should be noted, that even a small automatic film processor requires a separate, totally reliable electric supply for 3–4 kW, access to plenty of clean water, and well trained personnel for daily use and maintenance.

Manual film processing

Manual processing requires more precision and attention from the darkroom technician than does automatic film processing, especially if the room temperature is high and the ventilation is poor.

A detailed description of the activities in and around the darkroom is given. It is anticipated that for the processing, a strict time/temperature control will be used, i.e. without visual control of the development.

For a detailed description of the management and maintenance of the darkroom (and examination room), the reader is referred to the WHO manual "Quality Assurance Work", Geneva 2001 (WHO/DIL/01.3).

Procedures for manual film processing in a staffed darkroom

1. Bring the exposed cassette from the through-the-wall cassette hatch to the dry bench.
2. Unload the cassette.
3. Mark the film with the name of the examined person, date and name of the hospital. NOTE: film marking can be made outside the darkroom with a photographic marker if cassettes with a protected area at the back are used. This may shift the marking job from the darkroom attendant to the radiographer making the examinations, and will considerably improve the precision of the developing procedure.
4. Mount the film into a stainless steel frame of correct size.
5. Put the frame with film into the developing tank, and move it up and down twice, eliminating air bubbles on the film, ensuring that the whole film gets in contact with the developer.
6. Start the darkroom timer (which must be preset for the appropriate developing time for the actual temperature of the solution). Normal range is 5 → 3 minutes at 19 → 23 °C. With special precautions, the temperature range can be extended to 25 °C, using 2 minutes for the development. Shorter developing times than 2 minutes cannot be maintained properly in routine work.
7. Reload the cassette with a new film and return the cassette to the through-the-wall hatch.
8. After 1/2 minute in the developer, move the film frame up and down twice and make space for the next film frame to follow this one. Do not check the film blackening!
9. After the predetermined developing time (2–5 minutes depending on the temperature), transfer the film frame to the stop/intermediate wash bath (without checking the blackening!). Move it up and down two or three times during 1/2 minute, then transfer it to the fixing tank.
10. The fixing time is independent of the developing time, and is at least 3 minutes (for modern emulsions with low silver content), but preferably 5 minutes. Longer time will not damage the film. The film can be viewed in white light outside the darkroom after 3 minutes in the fixer, but should be returned to the fixer for another 3–4 minutes. Remember to put a lid on the developer tank before opening the darkroom door.
11. Transfer the film to the rinse tank, where it has to remain in running water for at least 30 minutes. Longer time will not damage the film. NOTE: the rinse water temperature should be close to the fixer temperature and not more than 27 °C.
12. Films are best dried (in their hangers) in a drying cabinet with forced ventilation, located outside the darkroom. If the air is heated, a thermostat must control the temperature so that it does not exceed 35 °C. If there is no drying cabinet, make sure that films hang where there is no dust and that the hangers are firmly fixed so they do not fall onto the ground. It is very difficult to remove dirt from a film, and scratches cannot be removed. If films in hangers are sent away from the darkroom, rinse them in the wash-tank for a few minutes when they are returned. Then dry them.

Technical background for the WHIS-RAD equipment

As stated in Chapter 1, the present manual is primarily adapted to the WHIS-RAD equipment (The World Health Imaging System for Radiology), but with appropriate modification the manual can be used with any type of adequate radiographic equipment.

In the present chapter, the technical requirements for the WHIS-RAD equipment, optimized for all general radiographic examinations, are given. Thus, equipments suitable for special procedures and fluoroscopy will not be mentioned.

General considerations

For the creation of an x-ray unit, designed to be successfully used for all general radiographic examinations, the demands on the construction optimizations and limitations together should produce excellent image quality with a low radiation dose. The most crucial points are the completely fixed imaging geometry from tube to casette holder with fixed grid, and the choice of appropriate generator and tube in combination with appropriate film-screen combinations.

After many years of discussions and trials, a WHO expert group delivered the solution named WHIS-RAD, fulfilling the demands. The special "prone question mark" design of the stand (see figure 1) makes it possible to use it for all general radiographic examinations, and it is now successfully implemented in several thousands small and middle sized radiology departments around the world. (A detailed description and specifications of the WHIS-RAD are given in the WHO publication "Consumer Guide for the purchase of X-ray equipment", Geneva 2000, WHO/DIL/00.1 Rev.1).

The three most important influences on the design, to be discussed below, are:

1. Requirements related to the objects to be radiographed.
2. Imaging conditions affecting radiographic image quality.
3. The choice of a suitable x-ray source.

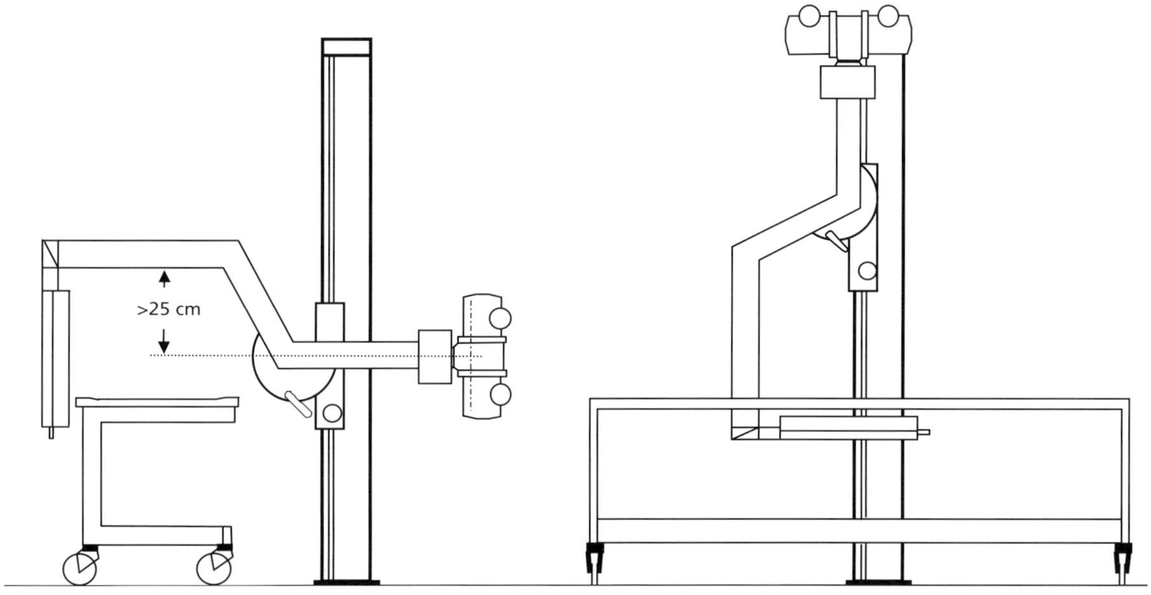

Figure 1 (from WHO/RAD/TS/95.1): The main features of the WHIS-RAD stand.

Radiographic objects

Three extreme imaging situations for which the equipment must be suitable:

The **very thin object** represented by the hand requires low tube tension in the range of 45–60 kV resulting in high contrast, small geometric magnification giving negligible geometric unsharpness, and an image recording medium with excellent detail resolution.

The **very dense object**, represented by the lateral view of the lumbosacral junction, may have a density corresponding to as much as 30 cm of water. The choice of kV-values becomes a compromise between required film density and acceptable image contrast. In practice the tube tension should not be more than 90 kV with less than 4% ripple.

A long focus-film distance or a very small focal spot is needed; an FFD of 120 cm or more in combination with a focal spot of 1 mm or less is acceptable. The screen-film combination will be a compromise between recording system speed (sensitivity) and detail resolution.

The **chest** represents a unique imaging situation. High tube tension (kV) and very short exposure times should be used. In order to suppress the skeletal image, penetrate through the heart, and emphasize the contrast between air and soft tissue, the tube tension must be in the range of 110–140 kV with less than 4% ripple.

The image quality is improved if the radiation detector has low sensitivity in the lower end of the radiation spectrum. The high-kV technique is necessary to get suitable radiographic contrast and sufficiently short exposure times. The exposure times must be shorter than 50 ms.

The requirement for detail resolution is not very high in chest radiography. Most high speed screen-film combinations with a nominal speed larger than 250 cannot be used with standard focus-film distances of 150–180 cm, unless the X-ray generator can handle mAs-values down to 1 mAs with proper 26% increments between steps.

Imaging conditions

The radiographic image quality is influenced by **image contrast, detail resolution** and the **physical shape of the radiographic stand.**

Image contrast

Image contrast is influenced by tube tension (kV) and the ratio between primary image-producing radiation and scattered radiation.

The image contrast is primarily chosen by **selection of a suitable kV-value.** For bone the kV should be as low as possible.

In chest radiography the most suitable image contrast is produced between 110–140 kV (ripple <4%).

Image contrast is strongly influenced by scattered radiation. **If less than 1 liter of body tissue is irradiated, the scatter can be ignored.** When the tube tension is below 60 kV and less than 2 liters of body tissue are irradiated, e.g. a knee imaged on an 18×24 cm film, no action has to be taken against scattered radiation. In all other radiographic situations action must be taken to reduce the amount of scatter reaching the film; best done by interposition of a grid between object and cassette.

The choice of a grid is a very complex problem. **A grid with the ratio 10:1 usually is the best choice for general radiography.**

Modern grids with 40 lines/cm or more may remain stationary without disturbing the image, if the required image detail resolution is no more than 4 linepairs/mm.

Detail resolution

Detail resolution is affected by **geometric unsharpness, motion unsharpness** and **unsharpness originating in the image recording medium,** (usually a screen-film combination). All these factors are interrelated.

Geometric unsharpness is not easily defined in simple terms. A geometric unsharpness of 0.25 mm should not be exceeded. This corresponds to approximately 4 lp/mm.

In practice the magnification seldom exceeds 1.25 but may occasionally reach 1.35 times. X-ray tubes with a nominal focus size in the range of 0.8-1.0 mm are satisfactory in general radiography. The loadability should be 25–30 kW for 0.1 s and 30 kWs within 1–2 s.

Motion unsharpness is a type of geometric unsharpness which is directly proportional to the velocity of the moving object. The following exposure times should not be exceeded:

In the immediate vicinity of the heart	**10 ms**
In the chest in general (PA chest)	**50 ms**
For bone	**1–2 s**

Image recording medium. General purpose radiography is manageable using screen-film combinations with only two different speeds. For all radiographic images produced behind an antiscatter grid a resolution if 4 lp/mm is satisfactory. For images produced without a grid and with cassette size not exceeding 18x24 cm, the resolution should be at least 6 lp/mm.

Calcium-tungstate screens for blue sensitive film. Detail screens with a relative speed of 50 and a resolution of 8 lp/mm or more may be used for radiography of the extremities.

Fast or **HiPlus** screens have a relative speed of 200 and resolve about 3.5–4 lp/mm. They are used for all other examinations, including chest.

Modern green emitting intensifying screens for green-sensitive film are available in four different speed groups (nominal speed at 80 kV). (At 40 kV the speed values are halved.)

Fine	**speed = 100, res. = 8–10 lp/mm**
Medium	**speed = 200, res. = 6–8 lp/mm**
Regular	**speed = 400, res. = 4–6 lp/mm**
Fast	**speed = 800, res. = about 4 lp/mm**

The manual recommends the use of **Fine** screens for extremities, **Medium** screens for chest, and **Regular** screens for everything else.

Physical shape of stands for general radiography

It should be possible to X-ray a standing adult patient from shoulders to knee-joints. This requires that the **horizontal x-ray beam** can be used at a distance from the floor of 50–170 cm. Examinations of cervical spine and paranasal sinuses can be made with the patient standing or sitting. Note, however, that a proper skull examination should be done with the patient lying down. It must also be possible to x-ray a recumbent patient with a horizontal beam from head to feet.

It must be possible to x-ray a lying patient on a **radiolucent movable table-top** with **vertical x-ray beam** and with **a beam angulated up to ±30°** from the vertical direction. This must be achieved with no more than 1.3 × magnification of the structure of major interest.

It must be possible to examine the arm of a sitting patient with vertical x-ray beam, when the arm is at right angles at the shoulder and the elbow. This requires a horizontal cassette position 100–110 cm from the floor (e.g. on the top of the horizontal WHIS-RAD cassette holder.).

All these patient positions are often achieved by the use of two different examination stands. It is possible, however, to design a single stand to do them all. Such stands are the WHO-BRS/1985 Unit and the later developed WHIS-RAD Unit. These WHO specified units have a curved swivel arm with an FFD of 140 cm and fixed imaging geometry, but still the possibilities to angulate the x-ray beam ±30° from the vertical and the horizontal direction without excessive magnification. The gap between patient and film is only 25 mm in chest radiography, which at heart volume measurements is equivalent to 38 mm at an FFD of 150 cm or 65 mm at an FFD of 180 cm.

Fixed geometry guarantees:

1. Correct centering of the x-ray beam to the film,
2. Permanent centering of the grid, resulting in lowest possible visibility of the grid lines,
3. No variation in exposure requirements due to change in FFD. The long FFD allows tilted views in spite of the fixed geometry.

Angulation of the x-ray beam and variable film-focus distance in relation to the grid always results in longer exposure times and reduced image quality. A variable film-focus distance is also a common reason for erratic exposure!

X-ray source

The demands on the x-ray source can be concluded from what has been said about the dimensions of radiographic objects and about imaging conditions.

High-tension generator: *Single-phase 50/60 Hz x-ray generators or capacitor discharge generators with the capacitor in the high-tension circuit, cannot properly handle the extreme exposure requirements, represented by the chest and lateral lumbosacral junction.* Only 3-phase x-ray generators with **electronic switching in the high-tension circuit** and **multipulse x-ray generators, using high-**

frequency inverter technology, are capable of delivering the exposure factors required. Three-phase 50/60 Hz x-ray generators are disappearing from the market and are replaced by cheaper and more reliable multipulse generators.

Multipulse x-ray generators, using capacitors or batteries for energy storage, are now available to connect to weak or unreliable power lines or small petrol-driven AC generators.

X-ray tubes, used with the WHIS-RAD, must handle at least 25 kW for 0.1 s (= nominal rating) and half that for 1.6 s (= 20 kWs). The focus diameter must not exceed 1.0 mm (nominal value). Tubes which fulfill these requirements are available with focal spots in the range of 0.6–1.0 mm. If the long FFD of 140 cm is used for all examinations, the anode angle may be as small as 10°–13°. If the FFD is 100 cm, the anode angle should be 13°–15°.

Values of x-ray tube voltage. For didactic reasons the choice of kV-values is limited to a small number of fixed steps. In practice this leaves a satisfactory choice of radiation qualities for clinical radiography.

Recommended x-ray tube voltages

46 – 53 – 60 – 70 – 80 – 90 – (100) – 120 kV

NOTE: 100 kV is available for testing purposes only. *A larger number of kV-steps, or continuously variable tube voltage is not acceptable.*

The selected kV-value must not fall more than 5% from the initial value during a tube loading.

Selection of kV-values in practical use

- **46/53 kV for examinations of peripheral extremities (no antiscatter grid);**
- **(60), 70, and 80 kV for examinations of bone or iodine contrast studies;**
- **90 kV for very dense objects, barium "double-contrast", and children's chest;**
- **120 kV for chest (lung) examinations of adults and for barium contrast studies.**

Exposure changes (steps with 26% increments) between kV values available with the WHIS-RAD unit with blue and green emitting screen film system

kV	46		53		60		70		80		90		120
Blue steps		3		3		3		3		2		4	
Green steps		4		4		4		3		3		4	

Values of current-time product shall be indicated in mAs, chosen as decimal multiples and sub-multiples from Renard Series 10 (ISO Standard 497/1973):

R′10, the Renard Series 10

1	1.25	1.6	2	2.5	3.2	4	5	6.3	8

The range of fixed mAs values to be used in the WHIS-RAD

							0.5	0.63	0.8
1	1.25	1.6	2	2.5	3.2	4	5	6.3	8
10	12.5	16	20	25	32	40	50	63	80
100	125	160	200	250	(320)				

NOTE: It is not required that the entire range of mAs-values is available at all kV-values. Thus, it is acceptable that only 12 kWs is reached at 120 kV.

Comment: When the R'10 series is used, each exposure step has exactly the same size in the entire range (+26%). Film blackening should always be altered by mAs-variations, and never by kV-variations. Tube voltage (kV) variations are used to influence the image contrast.

Detailed exposure tables

Below, exposure values are summarized for all projections given in the previous chapters, and in addition values are given for additional projections that may be used in general practice.

Exposure factors

As stated in chapter 2, the presented exposure values are based on a standard WHIS-RAD installation, with a focus-film distance (FFD) of 140 cm, a fixed Pb/Al grid (with a ratio of 10:1 and 40 lines/cm focused at 135–140 cm) built into the cassette holder. When noticed, the cassette is placed outside the cassette holder, adjacent to the body part examined.

The exposure factors are based on a "reference man" with a height of 180 cm (6 feet) and a weight of 80 kg (175 lbs).

Note that the exposure factors as well are dependent on the brand of screens, brand of films, and the film processing. The values have to be locally adjusted.

Exposure factors for children are very difficult to give, depending on the different shape of children with the same weight or age. Approximate values are given but have to be individually adjusted.

The kV value will determine the contrast in the image.

The mAs value will determine the image blackening.

Film speed and cassettes

The nominal speed of the screen-film combination should be written on the cassettes.

In the **"green" system** (gadolinium-oxysulfide) the actual speed varies with the kV value, low speed at low kV values nominal speed at 70–75 kV and a little higher speed at higher kV values. In the manual, the used speeds of the screen-film combinations are 100, 200, and 400 for the "green" system.

In the **"blue" system** (calcium-tungstate and rapid yttrium-tantalate screens) the nominal speed is equal to the actual speed at any kV value. In the manual, the used speeds of the screen-film combinations are 50 and 200 for the "blue" system.

EXPOSURE TABLES "Green system"

Multipuls or 3-phase generator, Filter 4 (3) mm Al, Green screen–film system

"GREEN SYSTEM"	Recommended factors						Local factors	
	Cassette in- or out-side the holder	Film size	Nominal/ actual screen–film speed	FFD	kV	mAs	mAs	Notes
CHEST								
CHEST 1 PA standing	in	35x43	200/250	1.4	120	2		
CHEST 2 lateral,standing	in	35x43	200/250	1.4	120	4		
CHEST 3 AP sitting	in	35x43	200/250	1.4	120	2.5		
CHEST 4 lateral sitting	in	35x43	200/250	1.4	120	5		
CHEST 5 AP supine	in	35x43	200/250	1.4	120	2.5		
CHEST 1/3/5 PA/AP child 30 kg	in	24x30	200	1.4	90	2		
CHEST 2 lateral child 30 kg	in	24x30	200	1.4	90	2.5		
Chest lying lateral view	in	35x43	200/250	1.4	120	5		
CHEST 6 apical lordotic	in	24x30	200/250	1.4	120	2.5		
CHEST 7 lateral decubitus	in	24x30	200/250	1.4	120	2		
CHEST 8/9 ribs oblique	in	35x43	200	1.4	70	20		
CHEST 10 AP infant hanging	in	24x30	200/250	1.4	90	1.6		
CHEST 11 AP infant supine	out	24x30	200	1.37	70	2		
Chest bedside AP	Grid	35x43	200/250	1.4	120	2.5		6:1 ratio grid
Chest bedside lateral	Grid	35x43	200/250	1.4	120	5		6:1 ratio grid
Chest bedside flank	Grid	35x43	200/250	1.4	120	2.5		6:1 ratio grid
Sternum AP	in	24x30	400	1.4	70	25		
Sternum lateral	in	24x30	400	1.4	90	32		
Ribs lower	in	24x30	400	1.4	70	32		

"GREEN SYSTEM"	Recommended factors						Local factors	
	Cassette in- or out-side the holder	Film size	Nominal/ actual screen–film speed	FFD	kV	mAs	mAs	Notes
ABDOMEN								
ABDOMEN 1 AP supine	in	35x43	400	1.4	70	40		
ABDOMEN 2 PA/AP standing erect	in	35x43	400/450	1.4	80	25		
ABDOMEN 3 lateral decubitus	in	35x43	400/450	1.4	80	20		
ABDOMEN 1 AP supine child 30 kg	in	24x30	400	1.4	70	20		
ABDOMEN 2 AP standing erect child 30kg	in	24x30	400/450	1.4	80	12.5		
ABDOMEN 4 AP erect child 10 kg	in	24x30	400	1.4	70	10		
ABDOMEN 5 supine urography	in	35x43	400/450	1.4	80	32		
ABDOMEN 6 urinary bladder	in	24x30	400	1.4	70	100		
ABDOMEN 6 bladder+contrast	in	24x30	400/450	1.4	80	50		
Urography 15 kg	in	24x30	400	1.4	70	16		
ABDOMEN 8 pregnancy lateral standing	in	35x43	400/500	1.4	90	63		
ABDOMEN 9 pregnancy PA/AP	in	35x43	400/500	1.4	90	63		

"GREEN SYSTEM"	Recommended factors						Local factors	
	Cassette in- or out-side the holder	Film size	Nominal/ actual screen–film speed	FFD	kV	mAs	mAs	Notes
HEAD								
HEAD 1/2 Skull PA/AP	in	24x30	400	1.4	70	50		
HEAD 2 Skull AP 3 years	in	24x30	400	1.4	70	40		
HEAD 2 Skull AP 5 months	in	18x24	400	1.4	70	32		
HEAD 3 Skull semiaxial (Towne's)	in	24x30	400	1.4	70	40		
HEAD 4 Skull lateral	in	24x30	400	1.4	70	16		
HEAD 4 Skull lateral 3 years	in	24x30	200	1.4	70	8		
HEAD 4 Skull lateral 5 months	in	18x24	400	1.4	70	6.3		
HEAD 5 Sinus semiaxial or nose PA	in	18x24	400/450	1.4	80	25		
HEAD 6 Sinus and face PA	in	18x24	400/450	1.4	80	20		
HEAD 7 Sinus and face lateral	in	18x24	400/450	1.4	80	5		
HEAD 7 Nose lateral	in	18x24	100/63	1.4	53	8		Collimate to nose
HEAD 8/10 Mandible PA/AP	in	18x24	400	1.4	70	32		
HEAD 9/11 Mandible oblique lateral	in	18x24	400	1.4	70	6.3		

"GREEN SYSTEM"	Recommended factors						Local factors	
	Cassette in- or out-side the holder	Film size	Nominal/ actual screen–film speed	FFD	kV	mAs	mAs	Notes
SPINE								
SPINE 1/2 Cervical spine PA lateral	in	18x24	400	1.4	70	12.5		
SPINE 1/2 Cervical spine AP/lat. 5 kg	in	18x24	200	1.4	70	12.5		
SPINE 3 Cervical spine oblique	in	18x24	400	1.4	70	12.5		
SPINE 4 Cervical spine AP supine	in	18x24	400	1.4	70	12.5		
SPINE 5 Cervical spine lateral supine	in	24x30	400	1.4	70	12.5		
SPINE 6 Open mouth odontoid AP	in	18x24	400	1.4	70	20		Collimate
SPINE 7 Cervicothoracic reg. lateral	in	24x30	400/450	1.4	80	50		
SPINE 8 Thoracic spine AP	in	18x43	400	1.4	70	40		
SPINE 9 Thoracic spine lateral	in	18x43	400	1.4	70	80		
SPINE 10 Lumbar spine AP/PA supine/prone	in	18x43	400	1.4	70	50		
SPINE 11/12 Lumbar spine lateral	in	18x43	400/450	1.4	80	100		
SPINE 11 Lumbal spine lateral 20 kg	in	24x30	400	1.4	70	64		
SPINE 13 Lumbar L5 and sacrum AP	in	24x30	400	1.4	70	63		
SPINE 14 Lumbar spine L5 lateral	in	24x30	400/500	1.4	90	125		
SPINE 14 Sacrum lateral	in	24x30	400/500	1.4	90	100		
Lumbal spine bedside AP	G	18x43	400/450	1.2	80	25		6:1 ratio grid
Lumbal spine bedside lateral	G	18x43	400/500	1-1.2	90	63		6:1 ratio grid

"GREEN SYSTEM"	Recommended factors						Local factors	
	Cassette in- or out-side the holder	Film size	Nominal/ actual screen–film speed	FFD	kV	mAs	mAs	Notes
ARM								
ARM 1 Clavicle AP +/– 20°	in	24x30	400	1.4	70	12.5		
ARM 1 Clavicle AP +/– 20° child	out	18x24	400/250	1.3	53	5		
ARM 2 Scapula AP	in	18x24	400	1.4	70	12.5		
ARM 2 Scapula AP child	out	18x24	400/250	1.3	53	6.4		
ARM 3 Scapula lateral	in	18x24	400	1.4	70	25		
ARM 4/5 Shoulder AP	in	18x24	400	1.4	70	6.3		
ARM 4 Shoulder AP child	out	18x24	400/250	1.3	53	3.2		
ARM 6 Shoulder axial	out	18x24	100/63	1.25	53	25		
ARM 7 Shoulder AP sitting (fract?)	in	18x24	400	1.4	70	6.3		
ARM 8 Shoulder lateral sitting (fract?)	in	18x24	400	1.4	70	16		
ARM 9 Humerus AP/lateral	in	18x43	400	1.4	70	6.3		
ARM 10 Humerus AP sitting (fract?)	in	18x43	400	1.4	70	6.3		
ARM 11 Humerus lateral sitting (fr?)	in	18x43	400	1.4	70	12.5		
ARM 12 Elbow AP	out	18x24	100/63	1.37	53	10		
ARM 13 Elbow lateral	out	18x24	100/63	1.37	53	16		
ARM 14 Elbow AP (fracture?)	out	18x24	100/63	1.37	53	16/12.5		
Elbow plaster	out	18x24	400/320	1.37	60	4		
ARM 15/16 Forearm AP/lateral	out	24x30	100/63	1.37	53	10		
Forearm plaster AP/lateral	out	24x30	400/320	1.37	60	4		
ARM 17 Wrist PA/AP	out	18x24	100/63	1.37	53	6.3		
ARM 18 Wrist lateral	out	18x24	100/63	1.37	53	10		
ARM 19 Scaphoid	out	18x24	100/63	1.37	53	8		
Wrist plaster AP	out	18x24	100/80	1.37	60	8		
Wrist plaster lateral	out	18x24	100/80	1.37	60	12.5		
ARM 20 Hand AP/obliques	out	24x30	100/50	1.37	46	8		
ARM 21/22 Thumb AP/lateral	out	18x24	100/50	1.37	46	16		
Hand plaster AP	out	18x24	100/80	1.37	60	6.3		
Hand plaster lateral	out	18x24	100/80	1.37	60	10		
ARM 23 Finger lateral	out	18x24	100/50	1.37	46	8		

"GREEN SYSTEM"	Recommended factors						Local factors	
	Cassette in- or out-side the holder	Film size	Nominal/ actual screen–film speed	FFD	kV	mAs	mAs	Notes
LEG								
LEG 1 Pelvis	in	35x43	400	1.4	70	50		
LEG 1 Pelvis AP child 15 kg	in	24x30	400	1.4	70	25		
LEG 2 Hip joint AP	in	24x30	400	1.4	70	63		
LEG 3 Hip joint lateral no injury	in	24x30	400	1.4	70	63		
LEG 4 Hip joint oblique lat. injury?	in	24x30	400	1.4	80	80		
LEG 5 Hip joint lateral injury?	G	24x30	400/450	1.2	80	125		6:1 ratio grid
LEG 6/7/8 Femur AP/lateral	in	18x43	400	1.4	70	25		
LEG 6/7/8 Femur AP/lateral child	out	18x43	400/250	1.3	53	2.5-6.3		
LEG 9/10/11 Knee AP/lateral	out	24x30	100/63	1.3	53	40		
Knee plaster	in	24x30	400	1.4	70	20		
Knee standing PA/lateral	in	24x30	400	1.4	70	5		
LEG 12 Knee intercondylar space	out	18x24	100/63	1.1	53	32		
LEG 13 Patella axial	out	18x24	100/63	1.1	53	25		Collim. to patella
LEG 14/15/16 Lower leg incl. knee	out	18x43	100/63	1.3	53	32		
LEG 14/15/16 Lower leg incl. ankle	out	18x43	100/63	1.3	53	25		
Lower leg plaster	in	18x43	400	1.4	70	20		
LEG 17/18 Ankle joint	out	18x24	100/63	1.3	53	20		
Ankle joint plaster	in	18x24	100/80	1.3	70	16		
LEG 19/20/21/22 Foot AP/oblique/lat.	out	24x30	100/50	1.3	46	25		
LEG 19 Foot AP toes	out	18x24	100/50	1.3	46	10		
LEG 23 Heel semiaxial/lateral	out	18x24	100/63	1.3	53	20		
LEG 24 Heel semiaxial	in	18x24	400	1.4	70	32		
LEG 25 Pelvis and hip joint infant	out	18x24	400/250	1.3	53	5		

"GREEN SYSTEM"	Recommended factors						Local factors	
	Cassette in- or out-side the holder	Film size	Nominal/ actual screen–film speed	FFD	kV	mAs	mAs	Notes
CHILDREN								
CHEST 1/3/5 PA/AP child 30 kg	in	24x30	200/250	1.4	90	2		
CHEST 2 lateral child 30 kg	in	24x30	200/250	1.4	90	2.5		
CHEST 10 AP infant hanging	in	24x30	200/250	1.4	90	1.6		
CHEST 11 AP infant supine	out	24x30	200	1.37	70	2		
ABDOMEN 1 AP supine child 30 kg	in	24x30	400	1.4	70	20		
ABDOMEN 2 AP standing erect child 30 kg	in	24x30	400/450	1.4	80	12.5		
ABDOMEN 4 AP erect child 10 kg	in	24x30	400	1.4	70	10		
Urography (IVP) 15 kg	in	24x30	400	1.4	70	16		
HEAD 2 Skull AP 5 months	in	18x24	400	1.4	70	32		
HEAD 4 Skull lateral 5 months	in	18x24	400	1.4	70	6.3		
HEAD 2 Skull AP 3 years	in	24x30	400	1.4	70	40		
HEAD 4 Skull lateral 3 years	in	24x30	200	1.4	70	8		
SPINE 1/2 Cervical spine AP/lateral 3 months	in	18x24	200	1.4	70	12.5		
SPINE 11 Lumbal spine lateral 20 kg	in	24x30	400	1.4	70	64		
ARM 1 Clavicle AP +/– 20° child	out	18x24	400	1.3	53	5		
ARM 2 Scapula AP child	out	18x24	400/250	1.3	53	6.4		
ARM 4 Shoulder AP child	out	18x24	400/250	1.3	53	3.2		
LEG 1 Pelvis AP 15 kg	in	24x30	400	1.4	70	25		
LEG 6/7/8 Femur AP/lateral child	out	18x43	400/250	1.4	53	2.5–6.3		
LEG 25 Pelvis and hip joint infant	out	18x24	400/250	1.3	53	5		

EXPOSURE TABLES "Blue system"

Revised from WHO-BRS Manual of Radiographic Technique, 1986 in relation to the diameter—thickness—of the part of the body to be x-rayed.

For the WHO Basic Radiological System with a 10:1 lead/aluminium grid, using:

- **standard blue-sensitive x-ray film in aluminium cassettes with calcium-tungstate (blue emitting) screens, nominal speed 200 or 50,**
- **for CHEST as well green-sensitive X-ray film with medium gadolinium-oxisulphide (green emitting) screens (nominal speed 200).**

"BLUE SYSTEM" and "GREEN SYSTEM" Nominal screen-film speed 200		**kV**	**cm**	**mAs**	**Position of the cassette**
CHEST	Adults	120	16–18	1.6	In the cassette holder
			19–21	2	
			22–24	2.5	
			25–27	3.2	
			28–29	4	
			30–31	5	
			32–33	6.3	
			34–35	8	
			36–37	10	
			38–39	12.5	
			40–41	16	
CHEST	Children	90	8–11	2	
			12–15	2.5	
			16–17	3.2	
CHEST	Infants weighing up to 10 kg	70	8–11	2	Directly under the patient on the cassette holder
			12–14	2.5	

THORACIC CAGE

"BLUE SYSTEM" screen-film speed 200		kV	cm	mAs	Position of the cassette
RIBS OBLIQUE	Erect and supine	70	12–15	10	
			16–18	12.5	
			19–21	16	
			22–24	20	
			25–27	25	
			28–29	32	
			30–31	40	
			32–33	50	
			34–35	63	
			36–37	80	
			38–39	100	
			40–41	125	In the cassette holder
THORACIC SPINE LATERAL		70	16–18	32	
			19–21	40	
			22–24	50	
and			25–27	63	
			28–29	80	
CERVICO-THORACIC SPINE LATERAL		80	30–31	50	
			32–33	63	
			34-35	80	
			36-37	100	
			38-39	125	
			40-41	160	

THE HEAD

"BLUE SYSTEM" screen-film speed 200	kV	Size of skull	mAs	Position of the cassette
SKULL LATERAL	70	Small	25	In the cassette holder
		Medium	32	
		Large	40	
SKULL PA and AP SEMIAXIAL	70	Small	63	
		Medium	80	
		Large	100	
SINUSES and FACE PA	80	Small	50	
		Medium	50	
		Large	64	
SINUSES and FACE SEMIAXIAL and NOSE PA	80	Small	50	
		Medium	63	
		Large	80	
SINUSES and FACE LATERAL	80	Small	8	
		Medium	10	
		Large	12.5	
NOSE LATERAL	53	All	16	
MANDIBLE PA and AP	70	All	63	
MANDIBLE OBLIQUE LATERAL	70	All	12.5	

THE LEG: SPECIAL EXPOSURES

"BLUE SYSTEM" screen-film speed 50		kV	cm	mAs	Position of the cassette
KNEE INTER-CONDYLAR SPACE and PATELLA AXIAL		53	8	16	Directly under the knee or patella
			9	16	
			10	20	
			11	25	
			12	32	
			13	40	
			14	50	
			15	50	
HEEL SEMIAXIAL	Supine	53	6	10	Directly under the heel
			7	12.5	
			8	16	
			9	16	
			10	20	
			11	25	
			12	32	
HEEL SEMIAXIAL PRONE	Prone	70	6	25	In the cassette holder
			7	32	
			8	40	
			9	50	
			10	64	

ALL OTHER VIEWS

"BLUE SYSTEM"

Diameter (thickness) cm	Cassette on the table top (no grid) speed 50		Cassette inside the cassette holder (with grid) speed 200			
	46 kV mAs	53 kV mAs	70 kV mAs	80 kV mAs	90 kV mAs	120 kV mAs
1	8					
2	10					
3	12.5					
4	16	8				
5	20	10				
6	25	12.5				
7	32	16	8			
8	40	20	10			
9	50	25	12.5			
10	63	32	16	8		
11	80	40	20	10		
12	100	50	25	12.5		
13	125	63	32	16		
14		80	40	20		
15		100	50	25		
16		125	63	32	20	
17			80	40	25	
18			100	50	32	
19			125	63	40	
20			160	80	50	
21			200	100	63	25
22			250	125	80	32
23				160	100	40
24				200	125	50
25				250	160	63
26					200	80
27					250	100
28						125
29						160
30						200
31						250
32						320!